Essential Concepts in Anatomy and Pathology for Undergraduate Revision

Aida Lai

BSc

Student Doctor, Wythenshawe Hospital
South Manchester University Hospital Trust, Manchester

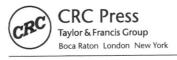

CRC Press
Taylor & Francis Group
Boca Raton London New York

CRC Press is an imprint of the
Taylor & Francis Group, an **informa** business

First published 2010 by Radcliffe Publishing Ltd

Published 2019 by CRC Press
Taylor & Francis Group
6000 Broken Sound Parkway NW, Suite 300
Boca Raton, FL 33487-2742

ISBN-13: 978-1-84619-413-9 (pbk)

Visit the Taylor & Francis Web site at
http://www.taylorandfrancis.com

and the CRC Press Web site at
http://www.crcpress.com

British Library Cataloguing in Publication Data

A catalogue record for this book is available from the British Library.

Typeset by Pindar NZ, Auckland, New Zealand

Contents

Preface

Anatomy and pathology are of major importance in our training as doctors. Yet the amount of knowledge to be gained in these two areas can seem overwhelming.

The purpose of *Essential Concepts in Anatomy and Pathology for Undergraduate Revision* is to help medical students to make the most efficient use of their revision time. This book contains the core basics that medical students need to grasp, and presents this information in the form of lists of key points for ease of reading and remembering.

This book draws on my experience both as a medical student and as an intern at various teaching hospitals. It is my aim to familiarise medical students in their pre-clinical years with the clinically relevant background information and knowledge of anatomy and pathology that are commonly encountered in end-of-semester exams. This book will help them to gain excellent results in those exams and prepare them for going on the wards. This is the book that I wish I had been able to use at the start of medical school.

Essential Concepts in Anatomy and Pathology for Undergraduate Revision is intended for quick revision of key facts. Students should consult reference books if more detailed descriptions or explanations are needed. Texts that I would recommend to supplement their reading of this book include *Netter's Anatomy*, *Robbins Basic Pathology* and *Wheater's Functional Histology* (for histological images). I sincerely hope that this book will be a useful addition to the medical student's bookshelf, and I would appreciate any feedback from readers to help to improve future editions.

Aida Lai
January 2010

About the author

Aida Lai completed her BSc (Honours) Medicine degree at the University of St Andrews. During her pre-clinical years, she served as clinical director of the Marrow Society. She has undertaken summer internships and placements in internal medicine divisions and surgical units at various teaching hospitals, and is currently undergoing clinical training at Wythenshawe Hospital in South Manchester.

Acknowledgements

I am most grateful to Dr Ng Wai Fu and Dr Chung Wai Ming for reading through the manuscript of this book and providing helpful advice.

I dedicate this book to Dr Susan Whiten, Dr David Sinclair and my family, who endured and supported me throughout the writing of it, and especially mom and dad, for getting me to where I am today.

1

Respiratory system

- **Nasal cavity**
  - Continuous with nasopharynx via internal nares
  - Roof of nose lined by olfactory epithelium (for smell)
  - Remainder of nose lined by respiratory epithelium (modified pseudostratified ciliated columnar epithelium)
  - Three shelves (superior, middle and inferior conchae; opening below shelves = meatus)
- **Conducting portion** (rigid conduits to warm and humidify air): ext. nose, nasal cavity, nasopharynx, oropharynx, larynx, trachea, bronchi, bronchioles, terminal bronchioles
- **Respiratory portion** (gaseous exchange): respiratory bronchioles, alveolar ducts (last part of respiratory tract containing smooth m.), alveolar sacs, alveoli
- **Epithelium lining trachea** = pseudo-stratified columnar epithelium (with goblet cells)
  - main bronchus = columnar epithelium (fewer goblet cells)
  - alveolus = squamous epithelium
- **Trachea**
  - Post. ends of cartilage connected by trachealis muscle
  - Begins at level of C6, bifurcates at T4/5
  - SS by inf. thyroid a. and bronchial a.
- **R. principal bronchus**: wider + shorter + more vertical (more common site for inhaled foreign objects to be lodged)
- **Bronchopulmonary segments** = pyramidal structures within lung lobes separated by connective tissue septum/partition (SS by own a. + drained by own veins + same segmental bronchus → can be resected surgically if disease occurs in a segment)

- **Pleurae**
  - Parietal layer: lines inner chest wall
  - Visceral layer: in contact with surface of lungs
  - Can be filled with serous fluid (pleural effusion)
    - (i) blood (haemothorax)
    - (ii) pus (empyema)
    - (iii) air (pneumothorax)
    - (iv) lymphatic fluid (chylothorax)
- **Lung** (costal surface in contact with costal pleura, and mediastinal surface in contact with mediastinal pleura)
  - (a) R. lobe (10)
    - R. upper lobe
      - 1 Apical
      - 2 Post.
      - 3 Ant.
    - R. middle lobe
      - 4 Lateral middle
      - 5 Medial middle
    - R. lower lobe
      - 6 Sup. basal
      - 7 Medial basal
      - 8 Ant. basal
      - 9 Lat. basal
      - 10 Post. basal
  - (b) L lobe (9)
    - L. upper lobe
      - 1 + 2 Apicopost.
      - 3 Ant.
      - 4 Sup. lingular
      - 5 Inf. lingular
    - L. lower lobe
      - 6 Sup.
      - 7 Medial basal
      - 8 Ant. basal
      - 9 Lat. basal
      - 10 Post. basal
- **Surfaces of lungs**:
  - Apex, diaphragmatic surface and costal surface
  - Blunt post. border + sharp ant. and inf. borders
  - R.: horizontal + oblique fissure (three lobes)
  - L.: single oblique fissure (two lobes)
- **Horizontal fissure**: runs horizontally at level of fourth costal cartilage → meets oblique fissure in mid-axillary line
- **Oblique fissure**: runs from sixth costal cartilage → T3 spinous process
- **Surface anatomy of lung bases**
  - Mid clavicular line: sixth rib

- Mid axillary line: eighth rib
- Mid scapular line: tenth rib
- **Arterial SS of lungs**
  - Pulmonary a. and v.
  - Bronchial a. (thoracic aorta) (anastomose with pulmonary a. in walls of bronchioles)
- **Venous drainage of lungs**
  - Bronchial v. (azygos v. and hemiazygos v.)
- **Lymphatic drainage of lungs**
  - Pulmonary nodes → hilar nodes → tracheobronchial nodes (tracheal bifurcation) → bronchomediastinal lymph trunks
  - Drainage from parietal pleura and thorax → axillary nodes
- **Innervation of lungs**
  - Pulmonary plexus (branches of sympathetic trunk + parasympathetic fibres of vagus n.)
- Lung apex extends 2 cm above ant. part of rib 1 (above clavicle) (covered by cervical pleura and suprapleural membrane)
- Rigid suprapleural membrane limits lung displacement during respiration
- **Pleural recesses** (separated by a layer of pleural fluid)
  - Costodiaphragmatic recess: between costal + diaphragmatic pleurae (lungs expand to this recess during forced inspiration)
  - Costomediastinal recess: between costal + mediastinal pleurae
- **Type II pneumocyte** produces surfactant (decreases surface tension, thereby reducing tendency of alveoli to collapse)
- Insufficient secretion in premature infants causes respiratory distress syndrome (RDS)
- **Attachments of external intercostal m.**
  - Origin: inf. border of rib above
  - Insertion: sup. border of rib below
  - Direction of fibres: ant. + inf.
  - Nerve SS: intercostal n.
  - Function: assist inspiration
  - Connected to ext. intercostal membrane ant.
- **Attachments of internal intercostal m.**
  - Origin: inf. border of rib above
  - Insertion: sup. border of rib below
  - Direction of fibres: post. + inf.
  - Nerve SS: intercostal n.
  - Function: assist forced expiration
  - Connected to int. intercostal membrane post.
- Innermost intercostal m. assists external + internal intercostal m.
- **Structures passed through when chest drain is inserted**
  - skin → superficial fascia → pectoralis major → ext. intercostal muscle → int. intercostal muscle → endothoracic fasica → parietal pleura
- **Accessory muscles of respiration**
  - Serratus ant.

- Pectoralis major
- Pectoralis minor
- Scalenus ant.
- Sternocleidomastoid
- Latissimus dorsi
- Needle for thoracentesis should be inserted near upper border of ribs to avoid disturbance of neurovascular bundle along inf. margin of ribs
- **Intercostal n.** = ventral primary rami of thoracic spinal n.
  - Gives motor SS to intercostal m.
  - Gives sensory SS to pleura and skin
  - Gives sympathetic SS to body wall structures
  - Branches:
    - (i) Collateral branch (runs on U. border of rib below)
    - (ii) Lat. cutaneous branch (divides into ant. + post. branches)
    - (iii) Ant. cutaneous branch (divides into med. + lat. branches)
    - (iv) Muscular branches
    - (v) Branches to parietal pleura
- **Intercostal a. + v.**
  - Ant. intercostal a. (1–7 from int. thoracic a., and 8–10 from musculophrenic a.)
  - Post. intercostal a. (1–2 from branch of costocervical trunk of second part of subclavian a., and 3–11 from subcostal a. of aorta)
  - Ant. intercostal v. (venae comitantes of int. thoracic a.)
  - Post. intercostal v. (1 to BCV, 2–3 from superior intercostal vein → drain to arch of azygos on RHS, BCV on LHS, and 4–11 to azygos veins)
- **Root of lung**
  - Primary bronchus (lies most posteriorly), pulmonary a. (superior), pulmonary veins (inferior), bronchial a. + v., pulmonary n. plexus + lymphatic vessels, bronchial lymph glands
- **Structures at the hilum of lung root**
  - Pulmonary artery
  - Two pulmonary veins
  - Main bronchus
  - Nerves and lymphatics
  - Bronchial vessels
- **Sternum**
  - Sternal notch (T2/3)
  - Sternal angle (T4/5)
  - Xiphisternal joint (T8/9)
- Manubriosternal joint = secondary cartilaginous joint (limited movement) Xiphisternal joint = secondary cartilaginous joint
- **Structures at vertebral T4/5**
  - Sternal angle
  - Arch of aorta begins and ends
  - Trachea bifurcates
  - Sup. limit of pulmonary trunk

- Arch of azygos v. drains into SVC
- Ribs 1–7 = true ribs (attached to sternum by costal cartilages)
  Ribs 8–10 = false ribs (attached to costal cartilages of the ribs above)
  Ribs 11–12 = floating ribs (no ant. attachment)
- **Typical features of rib 1**
  - Short and flattened, with broad surfaces
  - Only one articular surface
  - Scalene tubercle
  - Groove anterior to tubercle caused by subclavian v.
  - Groove posterior to tubercle caused by subclavian a.
- **Typical ribs (ribs 3–9)**
  - Head (articulates with corresponding vertebral body + vertebral body above)
  - Tubercle (articulates with transverse process of corresponding vertebral body)
  - Subcostal groove (houses neurovascular bundle)
- **Atypical ribs**
  - Rib 2: much longer than rib 1
  - Rib 10: only one articular facet on head
  - Ribs 11 and 12: do not have tubercle/subcostal groove, have no ant. articulation
- **Terminal branches of internal thoracic artery**
  - Superior epigastric artery
  - Musculophrenic artery
- **Paravertebral gutters** = deep recess on either side of vertebral column formed by post. curvature of ribs
- **L. recurrent laryngeal nerve**
  - Branch of L. vagus
  - Passes between pulmonary artery and aorta (aorto-pulmonary window)
  - Can be compressed by presence of mass → vocal cord paralysis (hoarseness of voice)
- **Phrenic nerves (C3–5)**
  - Pass ant. to lung roots
  - R. phrenic n. runs along R. BCV, SVC, RA; pierces diaphragm at T8
  - L. phrenic n. pierces diaphragm as a solitary structure
  - The only motor SS to diaphragm
  - Sensory SS to fibrous pericardium, parietal serous pericardium, parietal pleura, central tendon of diaphragm → irritation of diaphragm can be referred to C4 dermatome, resulting in sensation of pain at shoulder tip
- **Vagus nerves (CN10)**
  - Enclosed in carotid sheath in neck → between BCVs and common carotid a.
  - Medial to phrenic n.
  - Pass post. to lung root
  - Form oesophageal plexus
  - R. vagus n. runs behind arch of azygos v., ant. to R. subclavian a.

- L. vagus n. runs on the LHS of arch of aorta
- Parasympathetic SS to thoracic + abdominal visceral organs
- Gives off recurrent laryngeal branches (RLN)
- R. RLN runs under R. subclavian a., runs up groove between oesophagus + trachea → larynx
- L. RLN runs under arch of aorta, post. to ligamentum arteriosum, runs up groove between oesophagus + trachea → larynx
- RLN give motor SS to laryngeal m. (except cricothyroid), sensory SS to mucosa below vocal folds
- R. vagus gives rise to post. vagal trunk
- L. vagus gives rise to ant. vagal trunk
- **Clinical significance of L. RLN**
  - Bronchial carcinoma spreads to hilar nodes of lungs
  - L. RLN is closely related to hilar nodes when passing under aortic arch
  - If L. RLN is damaged by tumour, persistent hoarseness of voice occurs
- **Thoracic sympathetic trunk**
  - 12 ganglia
  - Ganglia give sympathetic SS to heart, lungs, aorta, oesophagus and abdominal viscera (through greater and lesser splanchnic nerves)
- **Diaphragm**
  - Developed from septum transversum
  - Muscular part + central tendon (fused with pericardium)
  - Attached to xiphisternal joint ant., median arcuate ligament post.
  - Motor nerve SS: phrenic n. (ant. rami of C3–5)
  - Sensory nerve SS: phrenic n. (central part), lower intercostal n. (peripheral part)
  - L. crus arises from L1, 2; passes up → insert into central tendon
  - R. crus arises from L1–3; passes up → some fibres cross to LHS to form sling around oesophagus (prevent reflux of food)
  - Median arcuate ligament connects R. + L. crura (crosses ant. to aorta)
- **Diaphragmatic openings**
  - T8: IVC, R. phrenic n.
  - T10: oesophagus, vagus n., oesophageal a., oesophageal branches of L. gastric vessels
  - T12: thoracic aorta, azygos v., hemiazygous v., thoracic duct

  (can be remembered by the mnemonic of Voice Of America, which stands for Vena cava, Oesophagus and Aorta)
- **Thoracic duct**
  - Drains into junction of L. IJV and L. subclavian v.
  - Provides lymphatic drainage to entire body except R. UL and R side of head and neck
  - Begins as cisterna chyli below diaphragm → crosses to LHS at level T4/T5
- **Azygos vein**
  - Drains post. wall of trunk
  - Arches over R. lung root to drain into SVC

- Receives hemiazygos v. at T8 level
- Receives accessory hemiazygos v. at T7 level
- Other tributaries: lower 8 intercostal veins, R. superior intercostal vein, mediastinal veins
- Needle passing in layers between skin and lungs for biopsy of lungs:
  skin → subcutaneous tissue → serratus anterior → ext. intercostal → int. intercostal → innermost intercostal → pleural parietal memb. → pleural cavity → visceral memb. → lung
- **Borders of thoracic inlet**
  - T1, first rib, manubrium
  - Articulates with first c.c. (primary cartilaginous joint)
  - Structures passing through:
    - (i) subclavian v.
    - (ii) subclavian a.
    - (iii) inf. trunk of brachial plexus (T1)
    - (iv) IJV
    - (v) common carotid a.
    - (vi) trachea
    - (vii) oesophagus
    - (viii) R. + L. vagus n.
    - (ix) R. + L. phrenic n.
- **Borders of thoracic outlet (closed by diaphragm)**
  - T12, ribs 11 and 12, costal cartilages of ribs 7–10 (costal margin), xiphoid cartilage (level of T9/T10)
  - Structures passing through:
    - (i) IVC
    - (ii) Oesophagus
    - (iii) Aortic hiatus

Common pathologies

Causes of finger clubbing

(associated with diseases of the lungs, heart and abdomen)
- Lung cancer
- Pus in the thorax (lung abscess, bronchiectasis, empyema)
- Pulmonary fibrosis
- Congenital heart disease
- Infective endocarditis
- Cirrhosis
- Hepatocellular carcinoma
- Crohn's disease
- Asbestosis
- Oesophageal cancer
- Thyrotoxicosis

Tracheoesophageal fistula
- Congenital disorder
- Abnormal connection between trachea (mostly distal third) and oesophagus associated with U. oesophageal atresia + polyhydramnios (excessive amounts of amniotic fluid)
- Symptoms:
  - vomiting
  - cyanosis after feeding
  - frothy white bubbles in mouth
- Complications: pneumonia
- Management: surgical closure

Cervical ribs
- Fibrous band from C7 post. to rib 1 ant.
- (Neurological deficit) structures passing over rib 1 elevated → causes thoracic outlet syndrome
- (Vascular insufficiency) subclavian a. may be narrowed → post-stenotic dilatation → thrombus formation → emboli → acute ischaemia
- Anterior ramus of T1 stressed → weakness and wasting of thenar muscles

Common cold
- Usually self-limiting
- Caused by rhinoviruses (which irritate pharyngeal mucosa)
- Symptoms:
  - sneezing
  - fever
  - headache
  - sore throat
  - tiredness
- Complications: otitis media

Localised airway obstruction
- Normal pulmonary function tests
- Caused by:
  - lesion outside wall (lymph nodes)
  - lesion in wall (tumours)
  - lesion in lumen (foreign body)

Acute bronchitis
- Viral (more common)/bacterial (*Haemophilus influenzae*)
- Symptoms:
  - unproductive cough
  - fever
  - pleuritic chest pain

- wheezing
- Management: antibiotic treatments

Chronic bronchitis
- Also known as 'blue bloater'
- Chronic cough with expectoration for at least 3 months for at least 2 consecutive years
- Causes: smoking, exposure to irritants → hypersecretion of mucus
- Pathology:
  - mucous gland hypertrophy
  - squamous metaplasia of bronchial epithelium (increased risk of malignancy)
- Exacerbations: recurrent low-grade bronchial infections
- May progress to hypercapnia → hypoxia (reflex pulnonary vasoconstriction) → pulmonary HT (cor pulmonale) (RV failure)
- Symptoms:
  - productive cough
  - haemoptysis
  - dyspnoea
  - weight loss
  - barrel-shaped chest
- Signs:
  - cyanosis
  - oedema
  - crackles
- Investigations:
  - CXR
  - pulmonary function tests

Emphysema
- Chronic obstructive airways disease
- Also known as 'pink puffer'
- Irreversible enlargement of air spaces distal to terminal bronchioles with walls destroyed or distended → loss of elastic support causes collapse of bronchioles → airways obstruction
- Common types of emphysema:
  - (a) Centrilobular emphysema:
    - mostly seen in smokers
    - occurs in airspaces in centre of lobules
    - mostly in U. lobes
    - pathology shows respiratory bronchiolitis
  - (b) Panlobular emphysema:
    - occurs in all airspaces distal to terminal bronchioles
    - mostly in L. lobes
    - associated with α_1-antitrypsin (AAT) deficiency
- Smoking results in influx of inflammatory cells → elastase breaks down

elastin fibres and inactivates α_1-antitrypsin (anti-protease)
- Symptoms:
  - dyspnoea
  - hyperventilation
  - weight loss
  - over-inflated chest
- Signs:
  - anorexia
  - breathing through pursed lips
  - hyper-resonant on percussion
- Investigations:
  - pulmonary function tests
  - high-resolution CT scan
- Complications:
  - pneumothorax

Bronchiectasis
- Permanent dilatation of bronchi + bronchioles
- Common causes:
  - chronic inflammation causing increasing wall weakness
  - local obstruction (foreign bodies, extrinsic tumours, mucus)
  - enlarged lymph nodes
  - post-infections (e.g. TB)
  - cystic fibrosis
  - sarcoidosis
- Common causative organisms:
  - *Haemophilus influenzae*
  - *Staphylococcus aureus*
  - *Pseudomonas aeruginosa*
- Symptoms:
  - chronic cough with purulent sputum
  - haemoptysis
  - pleuritic chest pain
  - weight loss
  - intermittent fever
- Signs:
  - finger clubbing
  - crackles
  - wheezing
- Pathological features:
  - bronchial dilatation
  - fibrosis
  - inflammation
- Complications:
  - pneumonia
  - pneumothorax

- pleural effusion
- empyema
- meningitis
- amyloidosis
- Investigations:
  - CXR
  - pulmonary function tests
  - sputum culture
  - high-resolution CT scan of chest
- Management:
  - antibiotics if infection is present
  - bronchodilators
  - steroids
  - surgery (if advanced disease)

Pleural effusion
= serous fluid in pleural cavity
- Common causes: pulmonary infarction, TB, heart failure
  (a) Transudates = concentration of protein < 3 g/L
- Usually caused by HF/hypoproteinaemia
  (b) Exudates = concentration of protein > 3 g/L
- Usually caused by increased permeability of pleural capillaries due to infection/inflammation
- Symptoms:
  - dyspnoea
  - pleuritic chest pain
- Signs:
  - decreased chest expansion + dull percussion + diminished breath sounds on affected side
- Investigations:
  - CXR (blunt costophrenic angles) (confirmed by decubitus view)
  - ultrasound
  - pleural biopsy
  - CT scan
- Management: aspirate effusion

Empyema
= pus in pleural space
- Microscope findings: large numbers of neutrophils
- Usually caused by lung infections
- Symptoms:
  - rigors
  - weight loss
  - malaise
  - fever
  - SOB

- pleuritic pain
- cough with sputum
- Signs:
  - reduced breath sounds at affected lung base
- Investigations:
  - blood tests (increased WCC)
  - ultrasound-guided aspiration of pus
- Management:
  - antibiotics
  - suction tube inserted to drain away pus

Pneumonia

- Inflammation and consolidation of lung tissue due to infectious agents
- Community/nosocomial acquired
- Risk factors:
  - U. resp. tract infection
  - smoking
  - alcohol
  - uraemia

Atypical pneumonia

- Mostly due to *Legionella pneumophila*, *Mycoplasma*

Bronchopneumonia/lobar pneumonia

(a) Bronchopneumonia
  - Usually involves lower lobes, bilat.
  - Patchy areas of consolidation in lungs
(b) Lobar pneumonia
  - Complete consolidation of lung lobes
  - Mostly due to *Streptococcus pneumoniae*
  - Commonly involves pleura (may see pleural effusion)
  - Symptoms:
    - fever
    - cough
    - pain in chest
    - rigors
- Signs:
  - bronchial breathing
- Investigations:
  - CXR
  - sputum + blood culture
  - arterial blood gases
  - pulse oximetry
  - bronchoscopy brushings
- Complications:
  - lung abscess
  - empyema

- pleural effusion
- lobar collapse
- Management:
  - physiotherapy
  - antibiotics if infection is present

Pulmonary hypertension
- Can lead to RV failure
- Causes:
  - (a) Disease of the lung
    - COPD
  - (b) Diseases of vessels in the lung
    - primary pulmonary hypertension
    - multiple pulmonary a. stenosis
    - schistosomiasis
  - (c) Diseases of the heart
    - LV failure
    - mitral stenosis
  - (d) Musculoskeletal disorders
    - poliomyelitis
    - kyphoscoliosis
- Signs:
  - prominent 'V' wave in jugular venous waveform
  - RV parasternal heave
  - hepatomegaly
  - ascites
  - peripheral oedema
- Investigations:
  - ECG (signs of RV hypertrophy)
  - CXR (enlarged RV)
  - echocardiogram
- Management:
  - treat underlying cause
  - physiotherapy
  - warfarin + oxygen for primary pulmonary hypertension
  - diuretics for RV failure

Lung abscess
- Necrosis of lung parenchyma
- Causes:
  - aspiration pneumonia
  - bacterial infection
  - bronchial obstruction (carcinoma/foreign body)
- Common organisms involved = anaerobes
- Symptoms:
  - pleuritic chest pain

- fever
- cough with sputum production
- malaise
- weight loss
- Signs:
  - decreased breath sounds
  - bronchial breath sounds
  - pleural rub
  - finger clubbing
- Investigations:
  - CXR (air–fluid level in circular lesions – cavitation)
  - blood tests (white cell count shows leukocytosis)
  - sputum culture
- Management:
  - postural drainage
  - antibiotic therapy

Severe acute respiratory syndrome (SARS)
- Believed to be due to corona virus
- Symptoms:
  - fever
  - chills
  - malaise
  - headache
  - myalgia
- Investigations: CXR (air space opacity)
- Management: antiviral therapy (ribavirin)

Acute respiratory distress syndrome (ARDS)
- Diffuse alveolar damage
- Life-threatening
- Causes:
  - Gram-negative septicaemia
  - aspiration of gastric contents
  - pneumonia
  - DIC
  - blood transfusion reaction
  - drug induced
  - high altitude
  - amniotic fluid embolism
  - intracranial haemorrhage
- Signs:
  - tachypnoea
  - hyperventilation
  - hypoxaemia
- Investigations:

– CXR (bilateral diffuse shadowing of lungs)
- Management:
  – mechanical ventilation
  – treat underlying cause

Tuberculosis (TB)

- Caused by *Mycobacterium tuberculosis* and related species
  (a) Primary TB – infancy and childhood
    – Fine discrete nodular opacities in middle lobe, lower lobes and anterior segment of upper lobes
    – Hilar lymphadenopathy
    – Ghon's lesion = calcified lung lesion/scar
  (b) Reactivated TB – adolescence and adulthood
    – Infiltration with cavitation due to caseous necrosis
    – Mostly in apical and posterior segments of upper lobe
  (c) Miliary TB = widespread dissemination of TB due to bloodstream spread with multiple nodules present on CXR
- Symptoms:
  – SOB
  – fever
  – chronic productive cough
  – weight loss
  – malaise
  – haemoptysis
  – wheeze
- Investigations:
  – bronchoalveolar lavage
  – polymerase chain reaction (PCR) on respiratory samples
  – sputum culture and staining for acid-fast bacilli (Ziehl–Neelsen stain)
  – CXR (cavitating apical lesions – reactivated TB)
  – Mantoux test (tuberculin skin test)
  – CT scan
  – lung biopsy
- Pathological features:
  – caseating granulomas
  – primary infection: Ghon complex (infected calcified focus in lung plus associated lymph node), usually in mid zone
  – post-primary infection, usually in apex
- Complications:
  – cor pulmonale
  – fibrosis of lung
  – obstructive airways disease
  – bronchiectasis
  – amyloidosis
- Management: 6 months of rifampicin + isoniazid and pyrazinamide + ethambutol for initial 2 months

- Prevention: BCG vaccination

Legionnaire's disease
- Caused by *Legionella pneumophila* bacteria (Gram negative)
- Symptoms:
  - anorexia
  - headache
  - fever with rigor
  - malaise
  - non-productive cough
  - abdominal pain
  - diarrhoea
- Investigations:
  - blood tests
  - CXR
  - urine antigen test
- Management: erythromycin

Atopic asthma (reversible condition)
- Chronic inflammation of airways due to increased irritability and consequent widespread narrowing of bronchial tree
- Type I hypersensitivity condition
- Associated with family history
- Triggering factors:
  - cold air
  - air pollution
  - pollens
  - smoke
  - dust mites
  - fungal spores
  - viral infections
  - exercise
- 'Morning dip' in peak expiratory flow readings
- Pathology findings:
  - mucus plugging + inflammed bronchi
  - mucous gland + bronchial smooth muscle wall hypertrophy
- Symptoms:
  - dyspnoea
  - cough
- Signs:
  - nasal flaring
  - wheezing
  - cyanosis (severe cases)
- Investigations:
  - pulmonary function tests (reduced peak expiratory flow)
  - arterial blood gases

- CXR
- blood tests (eosinophilia)
- Management:
  - metered-dose inhaler
  - bronchodilators

Chronic obstructive pulmonary disease (COPD)
- Coexistence of chronic bronchitis + emphysema
- Most common cause: smoking
- Risk factors:
  - smoking
  - family history
  - chronic exposure to pollutants
  - recurrent respiratory infections
  - hyperactive airway
  - α_1-antitrypsin deficiency
- Symptoms:
  - breathing through pursed lips
  - use of accessory muscles
  - intercostal indrawing during inspiration
- Signs:
  - central cyanosis
  - reduced breath sounds during auscultation
- Investigations:
  - pulmonary function tests
  - spirometry
- Complications:
  - respiratory failure
  - cor pulmonale
- Management:
  - antibiotics (acute exacerbations)
  - smoking cessation
  - corticosteroids (beclomethasone)
  - bronchodilators
  - surgery

Atelectasis
= collapse of the lung

Compression atelectasis
- Due to fluid/air in pleural cavity
- Most commonly caused by congestive heart failure

Resorption atelectasis
- Due to obstruction in airway

Lung cancer (bronchogenic carcinoma)
- Causes:
  - smoking
  - asbestos
  - pulmonary fibrosis (adenocarcinoma)
- Microscopic features

Non-small-cell carcinoma (85%)
(a) Squamous-cell carcinoma
  - Mostly hilar
  - Mostly necrotic
  - Produces atelectasis
(b) Adenocarcinoma
  - Most common
  - Arises from glandular cells
  - Associated with pulmonary fibrosis (usually asbestos)
(c) Large-cell undifferentiated carcinoma
  - Least common
  - Strongly associated with smoking
  - Aggressive tumours

Small-cell carcinoma (15%)
- Smoker
- Early metastasis → worse prognosis
- Neuroendocrine tumour
- May secrete hormones, especially ADH/ACTH
- Made up of small blue cells
- Mitotic figures high
- Symptoms:
  - cough
  - haemoptysis
  - dyspnoea
  - epilepsy (cerebral metastases)
  - bone fracture (bone metastases)
  - finger clubbing
  - weight loss
  - cachexia
- Investigations:
  - CXR
  - sputum cytology
  - CT scan of thorax (staging)
  - bronchoscopy
- Complications:
  - spread to hilar nodes, tracheobronchial nodes and pleura
  - metastasises to liver, brain and bone
- Management:
  - surgery (non-small-cell carcinoma)

– chemotherapy (small-cell carinoma)

Secondary lung tumours
• More common than primary tumours
• Most common primary sites are colon and breast

Pancoast's syndrome
= tumour near apex of lung
• Affects T1 sympathetic ganglion (lies on the head of rib 1; also known as stellate ganglion)
• Usually squamous-cell carcinoma
• Symptoms:
    – ipsilateral Horner's syndrome
    – atrophy of hand and arm muscles (infiltration of C8–T2 brachial plexus)
• Symptoms of Horner's syndrome:
    – hemianhidrosis (absent sympathetic SS)
    – ptosis (partial paralysis of levator palpebrae superioris)
    – pupillary miosis (unopposed parasympathetic SS)
    – enophthalmos (paralysis of SS to orbitalis m.)

Malignant mesothelioma
• Neoplasm of visceral pleura
• Poor prognosis
• Risk factors:
    – asbestos exposure
    – smoking
• May present 30 years or more after exposure
• Symptoms:
    – local: pleuritic pain, dyspnoea
    – diffuse: chest pain, weight loss, malaise
• Signs: pleural effusion
• Investigations:
    – CXR
    – CT
    – pleural biopsy

Pneumothorax
= air in pleural cavity

Tension pneumothorax
= opening into pleura allowing entrance of air into pleural cavity during inspiration, but air cannot escape during expiration → P in pleural cavity builds up → mediastinum is shifted to opposite side and lung will be collapsed
• Surgical emergency
• Symptoms:
    – severe dyspnoea

- tachypnoea
- severe tachycardia
- sudden onset of pleuritic pain
- cyanosis
- Signs:
  - tracheal deviation from affected side
  - no thoracic movement + hyper-resonant + reduced breath sounds on affected side
- Management:
  - needle thoracostomy in second ICS mid-clavicular line on affected side → intercostal drain in fifth ICS midaxillary line
- Diagnosis confirmed by CXR (elevated diaphragm on affected side, mediastinal shift to opposite side)

Spontaneous pneumothorax
= spontaneous occurrence of gas in pleural cavity
- Mostly occurs in tall, thin people
- Symptoms:
  - sudden-onset pleuritic chest pain
- Signs:
  - reduced chest expansion and reduced breath sounds on affected side
- Diagnosis confirmed by CXR (elevated diaphragm on affected side)
- Management: aspiration if condition is severe

Pulmonary embolism (PE)
- Causes:
  - dislodged thrombus from deep vein thrombosis
  - immobility/disability
  - recent surgery (hip/knee replacement)
  - recent stroke/MI
  - pregnancy
  - coagulopathy
- Results in respiratory compromise + haemodynamic compromise
- Symptoms:
  - dyspnoea
  - acute onset of pleuritic chest pain
  - acute shortness of breath
  - haemoptysis
- Signs:
  - tachycardia
  - cyanosis
  - tachypnoea
  - pleural rub
  - raised JVP
  - pleural effusion
  - shock

- Investigations:
  - arterial blood gases (hypoxaemia in cases of massive pulmonary emboli)
  - CXR (wedge-shaped infiltrate)
  - ECG (S1Q3T3)
  - D-dimers (fibrin degradation product)
  - V/Q (ventilation–perfusion) scan
  - CT scan with IV contrast
  - MRI (pulmonary angiogram)
- Management:
  - high-flow oxygen
  - low-molecular-weight heparin (LMWH)/oral warfarin (anticoagulation)

Pulmonary oedema
(a) Due to change in Starling forces (transudate)
- Increased hydrostatic pressure (cardiogenic causes: left-sided HF, mitral stenosis)
- Reduced oncotic pressure (cirrhosis, nephrotic syndrome)

(b) Due to alveolar damage (exudate)
- Aspiration, infection, high altitude, drugs
- Symptoms:
  - dyspnoea
  - tachypnoea
  - orthopnoea
  - pink frothy sputum
- Investigations:
  - CXR
  - ECG (signs of MI)
  - U&Es
  - ABG (arterial blood gases)
- Management: sit patient up → give O_2 → IV frusemide (change to oral frusemide if stable)

Sarcoidosis
- Multi-system disorder
- Commonly involves lungs
- Characterised by non-caseating epithelioid granuloma
- Symptoms:
  - skin plaques
  - renal stones
- Systemic manifestations:
  - lymphadenopathy
  - enlargement of parotid gland
  - splenomegaly
  - osteoporosis
  - interstitial lung disease
  - cardiac arrhythmia

- – erythema nodosum
- Investigations:
  - – serum calcium levels (raised)
  - – CXR
  - – bronchoscopy
  - – bronchoalveolar lavage
- Management: prednisolone therapy

2

Cardiovascular system

- **Wall of blood vessels**
  - (a) tunica intima
    - – innermost endothelium
    - – sub. endothelial layer
    - – int. elastic lamina
  - (b) tunica media
    - – thickest layer
    - – smooth m. fibres
    - – elastic lamina
    - – ext. elastic lamina
  - (c) tunica adventitia
    - – outermost layer
      collagen and elastic fibres
    - – vasa vasorum
    - – lymphatics
    - – n. fibres
- Arterioles: diameter less than 0.5 mm
  Metarterioles = smallest arterioles with same diameter as capillaries, but
  having a layer of smooth m. surrounding them
- Superficial veins lie in superficial fascia
  Deep veins lie along arteries, within fascial compartments in limbs
- **Histological features of striated skeletal m.**
  - – cross-striations (due to contractile proteins)
  - – elongated multinucleated cells
- **Histological features of striated involuntary cardiac m.**
  - – extensive branching of m. fibres
  - – desmosomes connecting muscle cells
  - – faint cross-striations

- – intercalated discs across thickness of m. fibres, gap junctions, oval nuclei
- **Histological features of smooth m.**
  - – no cross-striations
  - – spindle-shaped centrally located nucleus
- **Sup. mediastinum (between manubrium ant. and U. thoracic vertebrae post.)**
  First rib → T4/T5 level
  Contents:
  - – thymus gland
  - – R. + L. brachiocephalic v.
  - – SVC
  - – azygos v.
  - – aortic arch + branches
  - – int. thoracic a. + v.
  - – R. + L. phrenic n.
  - – R. + L. vagus n.
  - – oesophagus
  - – trachea
  - – L. recurrent laryngeal n.
  - – thoracic duct
- **Inf. mediastinum divided into ant. + middle + post. mediastinum**
- **Ant. mediastinum (between sternum ant. and pericardium post.)**
  Contents:
  - – thymus remnant
  - – mediastinal lymph glands
- **Middle mediastinum**
  Contents:
  - – heart
  - – ascending aorta
  - – SVC
  - – pulmonary a. + branches
  - – R. + L. pulmonary veins
  - – bifurcation of trachea + bronchi
  - – R. + L. phrenic n.
  - – R. + L. pericardiacophrenic n.
- **Post. mediastinum (between pericardium ant. and thoracic vertebrae post.)**
  Contents:
  - – oesophagus + n. plexus
  - – thoracic aorta
  - – thoracic duct
  - – azygos v.
  - – sympathetic trunks + splanchnic n.
- Structure post. to manubrium = arch of aorta
- Sternal angle = point where the second costal cartilage articulates with the sternum (level of intervertebral disc between T4 and T5)
- **Pericardium**
  (a) Fibrous pericardium

- attached to sternum ant. by sternopericardial ligaments
  (b) Serous pericardium
  - (parietal layer) in contact with fibrous pericardium
  - (visceral layer) in contact with heart
- **Heart**
  - from second rib to fifth ICS
  - enclosed between sternum ant. and vertebral column post.
  - surface in contact with visceral layer of serous pericardium
  - transverse sinus = recess formed by reflection of serous pericardium bounded ant. by pulmonary trunk + aorta and post. by SVC + LA
  - oblique sinus = recess formed by reflection of serous pericardium around veins on post. surface of heart
- **Principle of referred pain**
  Phrenic n. gives sensory SS to pericardium and pleura but also gives motor SS to diaphragm, so pain from pericardium/irritation of diaphragmatic peritoneum can be referred to the shoulder, since both afferents (visceral and somatic) synapse with interneurons running to the brain. (Brain cannot distinguish between the sensory distributions, so pain from visceral organs is regarded as somatic in origin.)
- **Ductus arteriosus**
  - Allows bypass of pulmonary circulation in fetus
  - Connects PT to inf. aspect of aorta
  - SVC → RA → RV → PT → ductus arteriosus → aorta
  - Becomes ligamentum arteriosum after obliteration
- **Ductus venosus**
  - Allows direct communication between umbilical vein, IVC (bypass liver) ductus venosus → IVC → RA
  - Oxygenated + deoxygenated blood
  - Becomes ligamentum venosum after obliteration
- Umbilical vein carries oxygenated blood from placenta to IVC → RA (becomes ligamentum teres)
- Umbilical arteries carry deoxygenated blood from fetus to placenta (become medial umbilical ligaments)
- **Characteristics of RA**
  - blood draining from SVC, IVC and coronary sinus (in post. coronary sulcus)
  - sulcus terminalis (at exterior of RA) extending from opening of SVC to opening of IVC
  - crista terminalis (interior of RA)
  - R. auricle anterior to crista (pectinate muscles)
  - smooth post. wall (where SA node is located)
  - sinus of venae cavae posterior to crista (where IVC and SVC empty into heart)
- **Fossa ovalis**
  = embryonic foramen ovale (allows oxygenated blood to bypass non-functional lungs before birth)
  - septum primum forms valve of foramen ovale

- **Characteristics of RV**
  - contains trabeculae carneae, some form papillary muscles → attach chordae tendineae which connect to cusps of tricuspid valves
  - infundibulum = smooth area leading to pulmonary valve
  - chordae tendineae prevent cusps from everting into atria when ventricles contract
  - septomarginal trabecula (moderator band) bridges lower part of interventricular septum to base of ant. papillary muscle → prevents overdistension of ventricles
- **Characteristics of LA**
  - wall contains valve of foramen ovale (prevents reflux of blood to RA)
  - four pulmonary veins drain blood from lungs to heart
- R. AV valve = tricuspid valve (prevents backflow to RA when RV contracts)
- L. AV valve = bicuspid valve (prevents backflow to LA when LV contracts)
- Aortic valve and pulmonary valve = semilunar valves (three cusps) (prevent backflow into ventricles when ventricles relax)
- **Cardiac skeleton**
  - Four rings surrounding AV orifices, aortic orifice and opening of pulmonary trunk
  - Maintain patency of openings and separate A muscles and V muscles
- Pulmonary trunk divides under aortic arch into R. + L. pulmonary a. (level T5/T6)
- Coronary arteries (vulnerable to arteriosclerosis → angina/MI)
  - (a) R. coronary artery (ant. AV sulcus) (usually dominant)
    - runs between R. auricle and pulmonary trunk
    - early atrial branch → SA nodal branch
    - R. marginal branch (SS lateral aspect of RA and RV)
    - post. interventricular branch (SS post. RV + LV)
  - (b) L. coronary artery (between pulmonary trunk and L. auricle)
    - LAD (left anterior descending)
    - runs in ant. interventricular sulcus
    - gives off diagonal coronary a.
    - SS interventricular septum with AV bundle, ant. walls of RV + LV
    - most commonly affected by atherosclerosis → can cause dysrhythmia if blocked
  - (c) L. circumflex artery
    - runs in coronary sulcus
    - gives rise to L. marginal artery
    - SS LA, post. walls of LV
- **Venous drainage of heart**
  (tributaries of coronary sinus)
  - great cardiac v. (ant. interventricular sulcus → coronary sulcus) (drains LA and LV)
  - middle cardiac v. (post. interventricular sulcus) (drains part of RV and LV)
  - small cardiac v. (accompanies R. marginal branch of R. coronary a.)

(drains part of RV)
  - venae cordis minimae (drains directly into chambers of heart)
- **Innervation of heart**
  - sympathetic n. through cardiac plexuses
  - parasympathetic n. through vagus n.
- **Conducting system of heart**
  - SA node → AV node → bundle of His → R. + L. branches of bundle of His → Purkinje fibres (subendocardial plexus)
- **Structures in superior mediastinum**
  - SVC
  - R. and L. brachiocephalic veins
  - arch of aorta (behind manubrium) + branches
  - R. + L. phrenic (between a. and v.) and R. + L. vagus nerves
  - L. recurrent laryngeal branch of L. vagus n.
  - trachea
  - oesophagus
  - thymus
  - thoracic duct + blood vessels + lymphatics
- **Structures in posterior mediastinum**
  - thoracic duct + lymph nodes
  - thoracic aorta
  - sympathetic trunks + splanchnic nerves
  - oesophagus + nerve plexus
  - azygos veins
- IJV + subclavian v. → R. + L. BCVs (post. to sternoclavicular joint)
  R. BCV + L. BCV → SVC (post. to first c.c.)
- Brachiocephalic trunk divides post. to sternoclavicular joint → R. subclavian a. + R. common carotid a.
- Ligamentum arteriosum: connects pulmonary trunk to arch of aorta
- Ant. surface of heart = RA + RV
  Inf. surface of heart = RV + LV
  Post. surface of heart = LA + four pulmonary veins
- R. cardiac border = RA (R. third → sixth c.c.)
  Inf. cardiac border = RA + RV (R. sixth c.c. → L. fifth ICS mid-clavicular line)
  L. cardiac border = LV (L. second ICS → L. fifth ICS mid-clavicular line)
  Sup. cardiac border = auricular appendage + great vessels (R. third c.c. → L. second ICS)
- Common carotid a.
  - bifurcation at level of sup. border of thyroid cartilage (vertebral level C5, 6)
- **Carotid sinus**
  - dilated part at beginning of int. carotid a.
  - baroreceptors that monitor changes in blood pressure
  - innervated by CNIX
- **Carotid body**
  - at bifurcation of common carotid a.

- – chemoreceptors detect changes in blood chemistry (mostly oxygen content)
  - – innervated by CNIX and CNX
- Dorsalis pedis pulse: between tendons of extensor hallucis longis and extensor digitorum longus
- Subclavian a. → passes over first rib → axillary a.
- **Parts of subclavian a. (divided into three parts by scalenus ant.)**
  - (a) First part
    - (i) vertebral a. (enters foramina transversaria of C6)
    - (ii) thyrocervical trunk
      - – inf. thyroid a. (closely associated with RLN)
      - – transverse cervical a. (anastomosis in scapular region)
      - – suprascapular a. (anastomosis in scapular region)
    - (iii) internal thoracic a. (divides into sup. epigastric + musculophrenic branches)
  - (b) Second part (behind ant. scalene muscle)
    - (i) costocervical trunk (SS first two intercostal spaces + neck region)
      - – deep cervical a.
      - – supreme intercostal a.
  - (c) Third part
    - (i) dorsal scapular a.
- **Branches of thoracic aorta (T5–T12)**
  - – oesophageal a. (SS middle third of oesophagus)
  - – paired bronchial a. (two on the LHS, one on the RHS)
  - – post. intercostal a. (SS third to eleventh ICS)
  - – subcostal a.

Common pathologies

Arteriosclerosis
= thickening and loss of elasticity of arterial walls, most commonly caused by atherosclerosis

Atherosclerosis
- Pathological characteristics:
  - – lipid deposit
  - – fibrosis
  - – chronic inflammation
- Risk factors:
  - – hyperlipidaemia
  - – HT
  - – smoking
  - – DM
  - – obesity
  - – increasing age

- gender (male)
- family history
- Pathogenesis of atheroma: chronic endothelial injury → increased endothelial permeability → macrophages engulf oxidised low-density lipoprotein LDL foam cells → smooth muscle proliferation → collagen deposition → formation of fibro-lipid plaque (lipid core + fibrous cap)
- Complications of atheroma: plaques can undergo ulceration/thrombosis, giving rise to emboli/haemorrhage
- Consequences:
  - infarction (e.g. cerebral infarction, MI)
  - carotid atheroma emboli may cause transient ischaemic attacks
  - aortic aneurysm
  - intermittent claudication (compromised blood supply to lower limb → pain on exertion)
  - gangrene (arterial insufficiency even at rest)
- Investigations:
  - coronary angiogram by CT
- Management:
  - statins

Iron-deficiency anaemia
- Causes:
  - (a) malabsorption of iron
    - hypochlorhydria
    - coeliac disease
  - (b) increased demand by body
    - pregnancy
    - menstruation
  - (c) blood loss
    - peptic ulceration
    - diverticulitis
- Investigations:
  - plasma ferritin levels
  - endoscopy
  - stool occult blood
- Management: oral iron supplements

Megaloblastic anaemia
- Defective DNA synthesis
- Cause: deficiency of vitamin B_{12}/folic acid
- Symptoms:
  - malaise
  - paraesthesia
- Clinical findings:
  - neutrophil hypersegmentation
  - raised MCV

  - raised LDH
  - reduced haemoglobin levels, pancytopenia in severe cases
- Causes of vitamin B_{12} deficiency:
  - hypochlorhydria (gastric acid helps to release iron from food)
  - pernicious anaemia
  - deficiency in dietary intake
- Causes of folic acid deficiency:
  - haemolytic anaemia
  - coeliac disease
  - pregnancy
  - lactation
  - oral contraceptive pill
  - deficiency from dietary intake
  - haemodialysis

Pernicious anaemia
- Autoimmune disorder
- Parietal cell antibodies in serum
- Symptoms:
  - pallor
  - glossitis
  - angular stomatitis
  - polyneuropathy
- Investigations:
  - blood tests (reduced serum vitamin B_{12})
  - bone-marrow aspiration
  - Schilling test

Haemolytic anaemia
= reduction in lifespan of red blood cells
- Usually autoimmune disease
- Consequences:
  - reticulocytosis
  - raised levels of unconjugated bilirubin in blood
  - splenomegaly
(a) Due to defect in red blood cell membrane
  - Hereditary spherocytosis
  - Autosomal dominant
  - Signs:
    - anaemia
    - splenomegaly
    - jaundice
  - Investigations:
    - blood film analysis (spherocytes)
    - osmotic fragility tests (less tolerant of hypotonic solutions than normal red blood cells)

- Management: splenectomy

(b) Due to enzyme deficiency in red blood cells
- Glucose-6-phosphate dehydrogenase (G6PD) deficiency
- Asymptomatic unless exposed to certain drugs or infectious agents

(c) Haemoglobinopathy
  (i) Sickle-cell anaemia
  - Autosomal recessive
  - Point mutation in gene coding for beta globin chain
  - Replacement of glutamic acid with valine at position 6 of beta chain
  - Symptoms:
    - anaemia
    - hyposplenism
    - vaso-occlusive crisis (occlusion of vessels in bone) → severe pain in bones
    - sickle chest syndrome (caused by vaso-occlusive crisis resulting in fat emboli from bone to lungs)
  (ii) Thalassaemia
  - Defect in synthesis of alpha/beta globin chains
  - Causes microcytic hypochromic anaemia
  - Types: α-thalassaemia, β-thalassaemia major (Cooley's anaemia), β-thalassaemia minor

Leukaemia
= proliferation of precursors of white blood cells
- Leukocytosis
- Infiltration of liver and spleen with leukaemic blast cells
- Causes:
  - exposure to cytotoxic drugs
  - exposure to ionising radiation
  - genetic causes
- Investigations:
  - complete blood counts and blood smear
  - bone-marrow aspiration
- Management:
  - supportive (e.g. red blood cell infusion)
  - chemotherapy
  - bone-marrow transplant

Acute myeloblastic leukaemia (AML)
- Eight types
- More common in adults

Acute lymphoblastic leukaemia (ALL)
- Philadelphia chromosome = t(9;22) translocation
- More common in children
- Management:

- combination chemotherapy
- allogeneic transplantation

Chronic myeloid leukaemia (CML)
- More common in adults
- Philadelphia chromosome = t(9;22) translocation
- Symptoms:
  - fever
  - malaise
  - weight loss
  - weakness
- Signs:
  - splenomegaly
  - anaemia
  - retinal haemorrhage
- Investigations:
  - fluorescein *in-situ* hybridisation (FISH)
  - bone-marrow aspiration
- Management:
  - imatinib (tyrosine kinase inhibitor)
  - allogeneic haemopoietic stem-cell transplant

Chronic lymphocytic leukaemia (CLL)
- Most common leukaemia in the elderly
- Symptoms:
  - fever
  - discomfort in splenic region
  - anaemia
- Signs:
  - hepatomegaly
  - splenomegaly
  - thrombocytopenia
- Investigations:
  - blood film analysis (raised lymphocyte count)
  - immunophenotype (CD20 + CD5 + B cells)
- Management:
  - antibiotics (for infection)
  - purine analogues (fludarabine)
- Complications of bone-marrow transplant:
  - graft-versus-host disease (GVHD)

Neutropenia
= reduction in number of granulocytes in blood
- Causes:
  - autoimmune disorders
  - viral infection
  - typhoid infection

- white-cell aplasia
- chemotherapy
- radiotherapy
- Symptoms:
  - malaise
  - chills
  - fever
- Management:
  - antibiotics

Multiple myeloma
= proliferation of neoplastic plasma cells in bone marrow
- Malignant plasma cells stimulate osteoclasts to erode bones
- Affects axial skeleton
- Associated with renal failure due to excessive light chain excretion causing nephropathy
- Symptoms:
  - anaemia
  - osteoporosis
  - bone fractures
  - bone pain
  - polyuria (due to hypercalcaemia)

Disseminated intravascular coagulation (DIC)
- Small-vessel thrombosis occurs
- Causes:
  - diffuse endothelial cell injury (e.g. burn)
  - trauma
  - sepsis
  - carcinomatosis (disseminated carcinoma) (e.g. pancreatic cancer, lung cancer)
  - amniotic fluid embolism
  - snakebite
- Symptoms:
  - peripheral gangrene
  - haemorrhage
- Investigations:
  - blood film analysis (fragmented red blood cells)
  - prothrombin time (prolonged)
  - blood tests (thrombocytopenia)
  - raised levels of D-dimers
- Management:
  - transfusions of platelets and red blood cells

Thrombocytopenia
= fall in blood platelet count

- Symptoms:
  - menorrhagia
  - epistaxis
  - skin bruising
  - purpuric rash
- Management: platelet transfusion
  - (a) Reduction in platelet production:
    - hypoplastic anaemia
    - megaloblastic anaemia
    - myeloma
    - leukaemia
    - alcohol
    - bone-marrow carcinoma
    - drug induced
  - (b) Increased destruction of platelets:
    - blood loss
    - drug induced
    - disseminated intravascular coagulation (DIC)
    - thrombocytopenic purpura
    - septicaemia
    - SLE
  - (c) Sequestration of platelets:
    - hypersplenism
  - (d) Dilution effect:
    - massive blood transfusion

Hodgkin's lymphoma (HL)
- Mostly originate from B cells
- Pathological characteristic: Reed–Sternberg cells (neoplastic giant cells)
- Symptoms:
  - fever
  - painless lymphadenopathy
  - pruritus
- Signs:
  - splenomegaly
  - hepatomegaly
- Investigations:
  - blood tests (raised ESR)
  - lymph node fine-needle aspiration/biopsy
  - CXR (mediastinal widening)
  - CT scan
- Management:
  - chemotherapy
  - radiotherapy

Non-Hodgkin's lymphoma (NHL)
- Mostly originate from B cells
- Commonly involve other organs
- Symptoms:
  - lymphadenopathy
  - fever
  - weight loss
- Investigations:
  - blood tests (raised ESR)
  - bone-marrow aspiration
  - lymph node biopsy
  - CXR
  - CT scan (staging)
- Management:
  - chemotherapy
  - radiotherapy

Hypertension (HT)
(BP = CO x TPR)
- Risk factors:
  - diabetes mellitus
  - smoking
  - dietary (too much sodium and too little potassium)
  - genetic predisposition
  - stress

Classification based on cause
(a) Primary HT (most common)
  - Idiopathic
(b) Secondary HT
  (i) renal D
   - most common cause
   - renal a. stenosis
   - glomerulonephritis
   - renal failure
  (ii) tumours in adrenal gland
      Conn's syndrome
   - phaeochromocytoma
  (iii) drugs (steroids)
  (iv) coarctation of aorta

Classification based on clinical features
(a) Benign HT
  - Slow gradual changes in vessels with chronic end-organ failure
  - Clinical features:
   - LV hypertrophy
   - hypertensive retinopathy

- chronic renal failure
(b) Malignant HT
- Rapid-onset changes in vessels with acute end-organ failure
- Clinical features:
    - HF
    - blurred vision due to retinal haemorrhages
    - haematuria
    - acute renal failure (fibrinoid necrosis of glomeruli)
    - intracerebral haemorrhage (stroke)
- Pathological feature of malignant HT: fibrinoid necrosis
- Investigations:
    - blood tests (serum cholesterol, glucose)
    - ECG
    - fundoscopy
- Management:
    - low-fat diet
    - limit consumption of alcohol
    - antihypertensive drugs (ACEI, calcium-channel blockers, diuretics)
    - statins
- Complications:
    - MI
    - stroke
    - renal failure
    - hypertensive retinopathy

Pre-eclampsia

= pregnancy-induced hypertension
- Due to imbalance of prostaglandin and thromboxane
- Extravasation of protein occurs
- Risk factors:
    - family history
    - diabetes mellitus
    - renal disease
    - hydatidiform mole
- Symptoms:
    - proteinuria
- Investigations:
    - blood tests (CBC, PT)
    - renal function tests
    - urinalysis
- Management:
    - bed rest
    - Foley catheter (monitor urine output)
    - in severe cases, vaginal induction of delivery
- Complications:
    - DIC

- liver dysfunction
- visual disturbances
- convulsions
- congestive heart failure
- haemolysis
- thrombocytopenia
- premature delivery
- fetal loss

Subclavian steal syndrome
- Obstruction of subclavian a. proximal to origin of vertebral a.
- Subclavian a. supplied by retrograde blood flow from vertebral a. through carotid a.
- Occurs when there is excessive demand from upper limb
- Symptoms: transient cerebral ischaemia
- Management: surgical bypass

Atrial fibrillation
- Common causes:
  - acute MI
  - hypertension
  - HF
  - hyperthyroidism
  - pulmonary embolism
  - COPD
- Symptoms:
  - dyspnoea
  - palpitations
  - chest pain
  - dizziness
- Signs:
  - irregularly irregular pulse
- Complications:
  - thromboembolism
- Investigations:
  - ECG (absent P-waves)
  - echocardiogram
  - thyroid function tests
- Management:
  - electrical cardioversion
  - anticoagulation

Dextrocardia
- Heart displaced to the RHS
- Can be associated with situs inversus (in which positions of the major visceral organs are reversed)

- Signs:
  - displaced apex beat to RHS
- Investigations:
  - CXR
  - ECG

Pericarditis

- Inflammation of serous pericardium
- Mostly caused by viral infection (coxsackie virus, herpes)
- Other causes:
  - bacterial infection (staphylococcus, pneumococcus)
  - fungal infection
  - acute MI
  - rheumatic fever
  - trauma
  - drug induced
  - uraemia
  - metastatic (lymphoma, breast cancer)
  - post-radiation
- Complications:
  - cardiac tamponade
- Symptoms:
  - central chest pain that radiates to the arms; pain relieved by sitting forward
- Signs:
  - pericardial friction rub
- Investigations: ECG (ST elevation, T-wave inversion, PR interval depression)
- Management:
  - NSAIDs

Myocarditis

= acute inflammation of myocardium
- Mostly caused by viral infection
- Other causes:
  - bacterial infection
  - fungal infection
  - idiopathic
  - drugs (penicillin)
  - sarcoidosis
- Pathological features:
  - diffuse infiltration of lymphocytes (viral infections)
  - diffuse infiltration of polymorphonuclear cells (bacterial infections)
- Symptoms:
  - fever
  - pain

- fatigue
- exertional dyspnoea
- palpitations
- Investigations:
  - raised levels of cardiac enzymes in blood
  - viral Ab titres in blood
  - ECG
  - PCR (viral RNA)

Infective endocarditis
- Endocardial infection leading to inflammation
- Usually in sites of underlying valvular/endocardial damage
- Risk factors:
  - congenital valve disease
  - rheumatic heart disease
  - prosthetic valve implants
  - septal defects
  - IV drug users
  - haemodialysis
  - immunosuppression
- Symptoms:
  - fever
  - malaise
  - anorexia
- Signs:
  - peripheral septic embolisation: splinter haemorrhage, Roth spots on retina, Osler nodes on soles and palms
  - finger clubbing
  - heart murmur
- Common causative organisms:
  - *Staphylococcus aureus*
  - *Streptococcus viridans*
  - coagulase-negative staphylococci (prosthetic valve patients)
- Pathological characteristic: vegetation of platelets and fibrin
- Investigations:
  - serum CRP levels
  - blood sample collection and culture within 24-hour period before initiating antibiotic treatment
  - transthoracic echocardiography (TTE)
  - transoesophageal echocardiography (TOE)
  - ECG
- Management:
  - IV antibiotics
  - surgery if infection is persistent
- Complications:
  - valvular incompetence

  - myocarditis
  - anaemia
  - glomerulonephritis
  - septicaemia (fever, weight loss)
  - septic emboli (stroke, infarctions)

Cardiac tamponade
- Fluid accumulates in pericardial space
- Causes acute heart failure
- Usually follows trauma to thoracic region
- Heart is constricted in confined space → venous filling is restricted → cardic output is reduced → shock occurs
- Symptoms:
  - fall in BP
  - shock
  - jugular venous distension
- Diminished heart sounds
- Investigations:
  - CXR (enlarged heart)
  - ECG
  - echocardiogram
  - cardiac catheterisation

Coronary artery disease
- Greater than 75% occlusion leads to ischaemia

Angina pectoris
= pain during physical exertion due to ischaemia of myocardium
(a) Stable angina (predictable pain when there is increased demand from the heart)
  - atheromatous stenosis in coronary arteries
(b) Unstable angina (unpredictable pain which may occur at rest)
  - obstruction of coronary artery due to plaque rupture + thrombosis
- Symptoms: retrosternal chest pain radiating to L. shoulder and arm, brought on by exertion
- Investigations:
  - resting ECG
  - exercise ECG
  - echocardiogram
  - CT coronary angiography
- Management:
  - sublingual glyceryl trinitrate (GTN)
  - coronary angioplasty
  - coronary artery bypass grafting (CABG) if no response to medications

Myocardial infarction

= area of necrosis of cardiac muscle caused by a sudden reduction in coronary blood supply (mostly thrombosis superimposed on significant atherosclerosis)
- Risk factors:
  - hypercholesterolaemia
  - HT
  - smoking
  - family history of CVS diseases
  - diabetes mellitus
  - oral contraceptive pill
- Symptoms:
  - central crushing chest pain
  - profuse sweating
  - SOB
  - dizziness
  - nausea and vomiting
  - pulmonary oedema caused by less efficient LV pumping
  - feeling of impending doom
- Complications:
  - arrhythmia
  - angina
  - HF
  - mural thrombosis (clot forms within ventricle)
  - cardiac rupture (causing haemopericardium)
  - ventricular aneurysm (due to stretching of newly formed scar tissue)
  - pericarditis
  - mitral incompetence
  - mural thrombosis
- Diagnosis:
  - ECG
  - cardiac enzyme levels (troponin I, T)
- Management:
  - high-flow oygen
  - aspirin
  - pain relief
  - beta-blockers
  - reperfusion: thrombolysis + coronary artery bypass surgery (CABG)
- Pathology: yellow rubbery centre of necrotic muscle surrounded by haemorrhagic border (4 days old) + infiltration by acute inflammatory cells → granulation tissue → fibrosis

Heart block
- First-degree block
  - lengthened PR interval
- Second-degree block
  - (i) Mobitz type

      – const. lengthened PR interval but occasional P-wave with no
        following QRS complex
  (ii) Wenckebach type
      – progressively lengthening PR interval until one P-wave not followed
        by QRS complex
- Third-degree block
  - complete dissociation between P-waves and QRS complexes

Aneurysm

= weakening of vessel wall resulting in dilation of lumen and increasing risk of
rupture

Abdominal aortic aneurysm (AAA)

- Usually occurs below branch to renal arteries
- Causes:
  - atherosclerosis
  - connective tissue defects
- Symptoms:
  - asymptomatic (in most cases)
  - pain in central abdomen/loin region
- Signs:
  - expansile pulsating mass
  - acute lower limb ischaemia (may occur)
- Investigations:
  - AXR
  - CT scan
  - ultrasound scan of abdomen
  - angiography
- Complications: (> 5.5 cm) rupture → blood loss to retroperitoneum →
  hypotension → shock
- Management:
  - smoking cessation
  - surgery (for leaking/ruptured aneurysm)

Syphilitic aneurysm

- Infection commonly caused by *Treponema pallidum*
- Usually affects ascending and descending parts of aorta
- Associated with aortic valve regurgitation

Dissecting aortic aneurysm (aortic dissection)

- Longitudinal tear in the intima and media of aortic wall
- Blood can enter media of aorta, splitting it into two layers
- Mostly associated with systemic hypertension, Marfan syndrome
- Risk factors:
  - hypertension
  - atherosclerosis in aorta
  - coarctation of aorta

- – trauma
- – iatrogenic (catheterisation of heart)
- Symptoms:
  - – acute onset of tearing pain in the chest, radiating to back/shoulder
  - – shock
- Complications:
  - – retrograde dissection to aortic valve → LV failure
  - – cerebral ischaemia → MI/stroke
  - – abdominal ischaemia
  - – lower limb ischaemia
- Investigations:
  - – transoesophageal echocardiography
  - – CXR
  - – ECG
  - – CT scan
- Management: surgical repair

Atrial septal defect (ASD)
- More common in females
- Mostly due to failure of closure of ostium secundum between atria (inadequate growth of septum secundum) → causes patent foramen ovale
- May present with right heart failure (L. to R. shunt) → RV hypertrophy → pulmonary HT
- Investigations:
  - – CXR (prominent pulmonary a.)
  - – ECG (R. axis deviation)
  - – echocardiogram
- Management: surgery

Ventricular septal defect (VSD)
- Most common congenital heart disease
- Defect at muscular septum or membranous septum
- Symptoms:
  - – dyspnoea
  - – pansystolic murmur and thrill (L. to R. shunt)
- Investigations:
  - – CXR (prominent pulmonary a.)
  - – ECG (RV + LV hypertrophy)
- Management:
  - – surgery

Patent ductus arteriosus (PDA)
- Connection between pulmonary trunk and aorta
- Usually closes within first 48 hours of life
- Usually occurs in premature infants
- Causes L. to R. shunt → blood flows from aorta to pulmonary a. → strains

heart and causes pulmonary HT
- Causes dilation of pulmonary a., LA and LV
- Symptoms:
  - failure to thrive
  - breathlessness on exertion
- Signs: collapsing pulse
- Characteristic continuous machinery murmur
- Investigations:
  - CXR (prominent aorta)
  - ECG (signs of LV hypertrophy)
  - echocardiogram
- Complications: congestive heart failure

Transposition of the great arteries
- Aorta arises from RV
- Pulmonary a. arises from LV

Coarctation of the aorta
- Congenital narrowing of the aorta near site of attachment of ligamentum arteriosum
- More common in males
- Usually distal to ductus arteriosus
- Formation of collateral circulation from intercostal arteries → dilation → erosion of ribs → notching of ribs
- Symptoms:
  - headache
  - epistaxis (due to hypertension)
  - dizziness
  - palpitations
  - claudication
- Signs:
  - radial femoral delay
  - bruits
- Complications:
  - LV failure
  - aortic rupture
- Investigations:
  - CXR (notching of ribs)
  - ECG (signs of LV hypertrophy)
  - echocardiogram
  - CT scan
- Management: surgery

Fallot's tetralogy
- Ventricular septal defect (causes systolic murmur)
- Overriding aorta (sits over junction between LV and RV)

- Pulmonary valve stenosis (obstructs RV outflow)
- RV hypertrophy (increase in size to cope with increased obstruction to RV outflow)
- Symptoms:
  - growth retardation
  - SOB
- Signs:
  - finger clubbing
  - central cyanosis

Aortic stenosis (AS)
= calcification of aortic valve → obstruction of LV outflow → LV hypertrophy
- Causes:
  - rheumatic fever (RF)
  - calcification of congenital bicuspid aortic valve
- Symptoms:
  - chest pain
  - breathlessness
  - syncope on exertion
- Signs:
  - slow rising carotid pulse
  - ejection systolic murmur heard in aortic area
- Complications:
  - LV failure
  - arrhythmias
- Investigations:
  - CXR
  - ECG (signs of LV hypertrophy)
  - echocardiogram
- Management: valve replacement with prosthetic valve

Aortic regurgitation
- Causes:
  - dilatation of aortic root in elderly and hypertensive patients
  - rheumatic fever
  - bacterial endocarditis
  - Marfan's syndrome
- Symptoms: dyspnoea due to LV failure
- Signs:
  - early diastolic murmur
  - wide pulse pressure
- Investigations:
  - CXR (enlarged LV)
  - ECG (signs of LV hypertrophy)
  - echocardiogram
- Management: valve replacement with prosthetic valve

Mitral stenosis (MS)

= calcification and narrowing of mitral valve → pulmonary hypertension →
R. heart failure
- Causes: rheumatic fever
- Symptoms:
  - dyspnoea (increased LA pressure → pulmonary oedema)
  - haemoptysis
  - hoarseness (increased LA pressure → impinges on RLN)
- Signs:
  - malar flush
  - L. parasternal heave
  - increased JVP
- Complications:
  - atrial fibrillation
  - systemic embolisation
  - pulmonary infarction
  - RV failure
- Investigations:
  - ECG (bifid P-waves)
  - CXR (enlarged LA)
  - echocardiogram
- Management: valve replacement

Mitral regurgitation

- Causes:
  - rheumatic fever
  - post-MI papillary muscle rupture
  - infective endocarditis
- Symptoms:
  - dyspnoea
  - orthopnoea
  - palpitations
- Signs: pansystolic murmur
- Investigations:
  - ECG (bifid P-waves)
  - CXR (enlarged heart)
  - echocardiogram
- Management: valve replacement

Congestive heart failure

- Failure to pump enough blood to meet metabolic demands of body
- Risk factors:
  - HT
  - previous history of CVS diseases

LV failure
- Low ejection fraction
- Forward failure
- Reduced tissue perfusion
- Causes:
  - systolic dysfunction (ischaemia)
  - increased workload (increased preload/afterload) (e.g. aortic incompetence, mitral incompetence, systemic HT)
- Blood flows backward → pulmonary oedema
- Symptoms:
  - fatigue
  - dyspnoea
  - paroxysmal nocturnal dyspnoea
  - orthopnoea

RV failure
- Backward failure
- Blood accumulates in venous system
- Causes:
  - cor pulmonale
  - RV infarction
  - increased preload (tricuspid valve regurgitation)
  - increased afterload (secondary to LV failure)
- Symptoms:
  - SOB
  - ankle swelling
- Signs:
  - raised JVP
  - pitting oedema
  - tachycardia
  - ascites
- Investigations:
  - CXR (enlarged heart, blunting of costophrenic angle from effusion, bat's-wing hilar shadow due to pulmonary oedema)
  - ECG
  - echocardiogram
  - cardiopulmonary exercise testing
  - cardiac catheterisation
- Management:
  - cardiac glycosides (digoxin)
  - diuretics
  - ACEI
  - beta-blockers
  - spironolactone

Restrictive cardiomyopathy

= impairment of ventricular filling
- Causes:
  - amyloidosis (most common)
  - idiopathic
  - sarcoidosis
  - haemochromatosis
- Symptoms:
  - fatigue
  - dyspnoea
- Signs:
  - increase in venous pressure with inspiratory effort (Kussmaul's sign)
  - fourth heart sound
- Investigations:
  - CXR (may have enlargement of atria)
  - echocardiogram
  - cardiac catheterisation
  - ECG (ST elevation, T-wave inversion)
- Management:
  - heart transplant (if severe)

Dilated cardiomyopathy (DCM)

= ventricular dilatation
- Causes:
  - idiopathic
  - autoimmune disease
  - persistent viral infection
  - thiamin deficiency
  - myxoedema
  - thrombotic thrombocytopenic purpura
  - SLE
  - glycogen storage diseases
  - thyrotoxicosis
  - diabetes mellitus
- Clinical features:
  - syncope
  - heart failure
- Investigations:
  - angiography
  - ECG (non-specific ST elevation, T-wave inversion)
  - CXR (cardiac enlargement)
  - echocardiogram
- Treatment:
  - diuretics
  - ACEI
  - heart transplant

Hypertrophic cardiomyopathy (HCM)
- Most common form of cardiomyopathy
- Hypertrophy of myocardium
- Autosomal dominant
- Diastolic failure
- LV hypertrophy
- Most common cause of sudden death in young individuals
- Cause: myocardial hypertrophy
- Symptoms: (classic triad) angina + breathless on exertion + fainting episodes (syncope)
- Signs:
  - systolic ejection-type murmur
  - double apical pulsation
  - pansystolic murmur
- Investigations:
  - echocardiogram
  - ECG
  - CXR
  - cardiac catheterisation
- Management:
  - beta-blockers
  - surgical excision of interventricular septum
- Complications:
  - atrial fibrillation
  - sudden death

Shock
Anaphylactic shock
- Reduced vascular resistance systemically
- Signs:
  - tachycardia
  - pallor
  - laryngeal oedema
  - facial oedema
  - vomiting
  - diarrhoea
  - warm peripheries
  - urticaria
  - bronchospasm

Hypovolaemic shock
- Reduced cardiac output
- Reduced perfusion of tissue in body
- Signs:
  - tachycardia
  - pallor

- oliguria
- irritability
- low JVP
- weak and thready pulse
- metabolic acidosis

Septic shock

= infection with systemic response (such as tachycardia) and hypotension that is responsive to administration of IV fluids
- Caused by endotoxin present in cell walls of Gram-negative bacteria which induces release of TNF → blood vessels dilate and body temperature rises
- Signs:
  - tachycardia
  - hypotension
  - nausea
  - vomiting
  - fever
  - warm peripheries
  - low JVP
- Investigations:
  - blood tests (white cell count, urea, creatinine)
  - blood gases
  - X-ray
  - ultrasound
  - CT scan
- Complications:
  - multi-organ failure
- Management:
  - give oxygen
  - give IV fluids
  - treat infection
  - control haemorrhage

3

Breast

- **Branches of int. thoracic a.**
  - ant. intercostal a. (SS ant. intercostal spaces 1–6)
  - ant. perforating a. (SS skin of thoracic wall + medial breast)
  - musculophrenic a. (SS diaphragm + ant. intercostal spaces 7–10)
  - sup. epigastric a. (anastomoses with inf. epigastric a.)
- **Arterial supply**
  - long thoracic and thoracoacromial branches from axillary a. (lateral)
  - vessels from internal thoracic a. (medial)
  - second to fourth intercostal arteries (perforating branches)
- **Venous drainage**
  - axillary v.
  - internal thoracic v.
  - post. intercostal veins → azygos system
- **Lymphatic drainage**
  - 75% drains into axillary lymph nodes (mainly ant. nodes)
- **Innervation**
  - ant. and lat. cutaneous branches of second to sixth intercostal nerves
- **Lobules** = secretory units of breast containing acini
  - Acini composed of epithelial and myo-epithelial cells
  - Acini → lobules → lactiferous duct → nipple
- **Attachments of pectoralis major muscle**
  - origin: medial half of clavicle, ant. sternum, costal cartilages 1–7
  - insertion: lateral lip of intertubercular groove (humerus)
  - nerve SS: medial and lateral pectoral nerves
  - function: adducts, medial rotates, and flexes humerus at shoulder joint
- **Attachments of pectoralis minor muscle**
  - origin: anterior surface of ribs 3–5
  - insertion: coracoid process of scapula

- nerve SS: medial and lateral pectoral nerves
- function: depresses shoulder tip, protracts scapula
- **Clavipectoral fascia**
  - pierced by cephalic v.
- **Attachments of subclavius muscle**
  - origin: rib 1 junction between rib and costal cartilage
  - insertion: inferior middle third of clavicle
  - nerve SS: nerve to subclavius
  - function: pulls clavicle medially
- **Attachments of serratus anterior muscle (forms medial wall of axilla)**
  - origin: upper 8 ribs + anterior intercostal membranes
  - insertion: medial border of scapula
  - nerve SS: long thoracic nerve
  - function: laterally rotates and protracts scapula
- **Long thoracic nerve**
  - course along lateral chest wall on serratus ant.
  - motor SS to serratus ant.
  - if damaged causes 'winged scapula'
- **Thoracodorsal nerve**
  - course on latissimus dorsi
  - motor SS to latissimus dorsi
- **Medial pectoral nerve**
  - lateral to lateral pectoral nerve
  - motor SS to pectoralis major and minor
- **Lateral pectoral nerve**
  - medial to medial pectoral nerve
  - motor SS to pectoralis major
- **Cooper's ligaments**
  - suspensory ligaments connecting deep fascia to skin of breast
- **Boundaries of axilla**
  - medial border: serratus anterior, ribs 1–4 + intercostal spaces
  - anterior border: pectoralis major, pectoralis minor
  - lateral border: humerus
  - posterior border: latissimus dorsi, subscapularis, teres major
- Six sets of axillary lymph nodes: lateral, anterior, posterior, central, infraclavicular and apical

Common pathologies

Fibrocystic changes
- Benign proliferative condition, influenced by hormones
- Mostly occurs between the ages of 30 and 55 years
- Most common symptoms:
  - breast pain
  - mass (due to cysts/adenosis)

- nipple discharge
- Investigations:
  - ultrasound
  - mammography
  - biopsy to exclude malignancy

Fibroadenoma
- Most common benign tumour in young women
- Smooth, firm, mobile masses with well-circumscribed borders
- Arises from loose connective tissue and epithelium
- Investigations: image-guided core needle biopsy

Paget's disease of the nipple
- Eczematous changes in the nipple
- Symptoms:
  - erythema and ulceration of nipple
  - burning sensation felt in areola
- Mostly accompanied by underlying malignancy (DCIS/invasive carcinoma)

Fat necrosis of breast
- Usually occurs after trauma to breast
- No malignant potential
- Pathological characteristics:
  - scar tissue
  - chronic inflammatory cells
  - lipid-laden macrophages
- Signs:
  - palpable mass

Breast cancer
- Risk factors:
  - female sex
  - increasing age
  - early menarche (< 12 years)
  - late menopause (> 55 years)
  - late first pregnancy
  - exposure to radiation
  - mutations of breast cancer susceptibility genes BRCA1 and BRCA2
  - high-fat diet, obesity, alcohol, smoking
  - oral contraceptive pill (OCP) and hormone replacement therapy (HRT), due to exposure to oestrogen

Non-invasive carcinomas (without invasion into stroma)
Ductal carcinoma *in situ* (DCIS)
- Histological changes found in small and medium-sized ducts
- Has potential to become malignant (invasive ductal carcinoma)

- Frequently unilateral
- Microcalcifications
- Investigations: core biopsy

Lobular carcinoma *in situ* (LCIS)
- Histological changes found in lobules
- Mostly in pre-menopausal women, usually incidental findings in biopsy
- Increased risk of breast cancer in both breasts
- Frequently bilateral

Invasive carcinomas
Histologically classified into several types (presented in decreasing order of frequency):
   (a) infiltrating ductal of no special type
   (b) infiltrating lobular
   (c) medullary
   (d) mucinous
   (e) tubular
   (f) papillary and others (5%)
- Haematogenic spread: can metastasise to bodies of thoracic vertebrae via azygos veins (no valves)
- Symptoms:
  - mass in breast
  - recent nipple retraction (due to Cooper's ligament traction)
  - nipple discharge
  - eczema around nipple (Paget's disease of the breast)
- Investigations:
  - cancer markers (CA15–3)
  - mammogram (spiculated mass)
  - breast ultrasound
  - MRI
- Management:
  - mastectomy
  - radiotherapy
  - adjuvant hormonal therapy
  - chemotherapy (for more advanced stages of disease)

Gynaecomastia
= presence of breast tissue in male
- Imbalance of oestrogen and androgen levels
- Investigations:
  - mammogram
  - ultrasound
- Management: surgical excision
- Causes:
  - drug induced (steroids, cyproterone acetate, spironolactone)
  - testicular tumour (secretes oestrogen)

- adrenal tumour
- cirrhosis (impaired steroid metabolism)
- idiopathic

4

Gastrointestinal system

- **Foregut structures**
  - oesophagus, stomach, liver, pancreas, gallbladder, first part of duodenum
  - arterial SS by coeliac trunk
- **Midgut structures**
  - second to fourth part of duodenum, jejunum, ileum, caecum, appendix, ascending colon, proximal two-thirds of transverse colon
  - arterial SS by sup. mesenteric a.
- **Hindgut structures**
  - distal one-third of transverse colon, descending colon, sigmoid colon, rectum, U. part of anal canal
  - arterial SS by inf. mesenteric a.
- **Layers of digestive tract mucosa (from innermost to outermost)**
  - mucosa (simple columnar epithelium → lamina propria → muscularis mucosa)
  - submucosa
  - muscularis externa
  - serosa
- **Salivary gland**
  - (a) Submandibular gland (mixed mucous and serous secretion), divided by mylohyoid muscle into:
    - (i) superficial part
      - larger
      - located in the neck
    - (ii) deep part
      - located in the mouth; main submandibular duct opens into floor of mouth on sublingual papilla at side of lingual frenulum
  - (b) sublingual gland (mucus secretion)
  - (c) parotid gland (largest, purely serous)

- **Relationships of parotid gland**
  - sup.: zygomatic arch
  - inf.: post. belly of digastric
  - post.: mastoid process
  - ant.: ramus of mandible
  - med.: styloid process
- **Structures within parotid gland (from superficial to deep)**
  - facial n.
  - superficial temporal v. + maxillary v. → retromandibular v.
  - ext. carotid a. → superficial temporal a. + maxillary a.
- **Parotid duct**
  - arises from ant. parotid gland
  - pierces buccinator
  - opens into oral cavity opposite U. second molar tooth
- **Oesophagus**
  - approximately 25 cm long
  - C6 to T12 (passes through hiatus in diaphragm at T10)
  - lined with squamous epithelium
  - relationships:
    - (i) ant.: trachea, LA, R. pulmonary a.
    - (ii) post.: vertebral column, thoracic aorta, thoracic duct
    - (iii) RHS: azygos vein, thoracic duct
    - (iv) LHS: descending aorta
  - cricopharyngeus muscle = upper oesophageal sphincter (narrowest point in whole GI tract)
  - diaphragm = lower oesophageal sphincter
  - points of constriction (where caustic substances may be trapped) = cricopharyngeal constriction, aortic constriction (arch of aorta) and diaphragmatic constriction
  - divided into three parts:
    - (a) cervical part:
      - striated m.
      - SS by inf. thyroid a.
      - venous drainage to BCVs
      - innervated by recurrent laryngeal n.
    - (b) thoracic part:
      - mixed striated and smooth m.
      - SS by oesophageal branches of thoracic aorta
      - venous drainage to azygos system
      - innervated by vagus n.
    - (c) abdominal part:
      - smooth m.
      - SS by L. gastric a. of coeliac trunk.
      - venous drainage to L. gastric v. and azygos system
      - innervated by vagus n. and sympathetic n.
      - lymphatic drainage: post. mediastinal nodes

- Nine quadrants of the abdomen:
  - RUQ (R. hypochondrium), epigastrium and LUQ (L. hypochondrium)
  - R. flank, umbilical and L. flank
  - RLQ (R. iliac), suprapubic and LLQ (L. iliac)
- Usual causes of RUQ pain:
  - peptic ulceration, gastritis, hepatitis, pneumonia (R. lung), cholangitis, cholecystitis
- Usual causes of epigastric pain:
  - peptic ulceration, drug-induced gastritis, gastric reflux, biliary colic, acute pancreatitis, abdominal aortic aneurysm (AAA), oesophagitis, angina/MI
- Usual causes of LUQ pain:
  - acute pancreatitis, MI, splenic infarction, gastric reflux, peptic ulceration, pneumonia (L. lung)
- Usual causes of RLQ pain:
  - diverticulitis, acute appendicitis, cholecystitis, ruptured ovarian cyst, ruptured ectopic pregnancy, pyelonephritis
- Usual causes of LLQ pain:
  - diverticulitis, pyelonephritis, ruptured ectopic pregnancy, ruptured ovarian cyst, pelvic inflammatory disease
- Layers of abdominal wall (from outermost to innermost): skin → Camper's fascia (superficial fatty layer) → Scarpa's fascia (deep membranous layer; fuses to fascia lata of thigh below inguinal lig.) → external oblique m. → internal oblique m. → transversus abdominis m. → transversalis fascia → preperitoneal fat → peritoneum
- Innervation of abdominal wall:
  ventral primary rami of T1–T6, iliohypogastric + ilioinguinal branches of ventral primary rami of L1
- **Attachments of external oblique muscle**
  - origin: lower 8 ribs to anterior half of iliac crest
  - insertion: xiphoid process, linea alba, ant. half of iliac crest, pubic crest
  - muscle fibre direction: inferomedial
  - nerve SS: ventral primary rami of T7–T11, iliohypogastric n. (L1), ilioinguinal n. (L1)
  - forms external spermatic fascia of spermatic cord; free border of aponeurosis forms inguinal lig.
- **Attachments of internal oblique muscle**
  - origin: lateral two-thirds of inguinal ligament, anterior two-thirds of iliac crest, lateral edge of thoracolumbar fascia to rib 12
  - insertion: lower three ribs, xiphoid process, linea alba, pubic crest, pectineal line
  - muscle fibre direction: superomedial
  - nerve SS: ventral primary rami of T7–T11, iliohypogastric n. (L1), ilioinguinal n. (L1)
  - forms cremaster muscle and fascia; forms part of conjoint tendon

- Neurovascular bundle lies between internal oblique and transversus abdominis
- **Attachments of transversus abdominis muscle**
  - origin: lower six costal cartilages, lateral third of inguinal ligament, anterior two-thirds of iliac crest, lateral edge of thoracolumbar fascia
  - insertion: xiphoid process, linea alba, pubic crest, pectineal line
  - muscle fibre direction: horizontal
  - nerve SS: ventral primary rami of T7–T11, iliohypogastric n. (L1), ilioinguinal n. (L1)
  - forms internal spermatic fascia; forms part of conjoint tendon
- **Attachments of rectus abdominis**
  - origin: pubic symphysis, pubic crest
  - insertion: costal cartilages 5–7
  - lateral margin = linea semilunaris
  - separated by tendinous intersections; midline separation by linea alba (xiphoid process → pubic symphysis)
  - nerve SS: ventral primary rami of T7–T11
- **Attachments of pyrimidalis**
  - origin: anterior pubis, pubic symphysis
  - insertion: linea alba
  - nerve SS: ventral primary ramus of T12
  - function: tense linea alba
- **Arterial SS of ant. abdominal wall**
  - sup. epigastric a. (one of the terminal branches of int. thoracic a.)
  - inf. epigastric a. (branch of ext. iliac a.)
  - deep circumflex iliac a. (branch of ext. iliac a.)
- **Attachments of psoas major muscle**
  - origin: lat. T12 to L5 vertebral bodies
  - pass under inguinal ligament
  - insertion: lesser trochanter of femur
  - nerve SS: ant. rami of L1–3
  - function: flex and laterally rotate thigh
- **Attachments of psoas minor muscle**
  - origin: lat. T12 to L1 vertebral bodies
  - insertion: pectineal line of pelvic brim
  - nerve SS: ant. rami of L1
  - function: flex vertebral column
- **Attachments of quadratus lumborum**
  - origin: transverse process of L5 + iliac crest
  - insertion: transverse processes of L1–4
  - nerve SS: ant. rami of T12, L1–4
  - function: laterally flex vertebral column
- **Layers of smooth muscle of stomach**
  - outer longitudinal
  - middle circular
  - inner oblique

- **Parts of stomach**
  - cardia
  - fundus
  - body
  - pyloric antrum (sphincter leading to duodenum)
- **Cell types in stomach**
  - chief cells: secrete pepsinogens (digestive E)
  - parietal cells: secrete hydrochloric acid + intrinsic factor
  - mucus-secreting cells
- **Arterial supply of stomach**
  - R. and L. gastric arteries (lesser curvature)
  - R. and L. gastroepiploic arteries (greater curvature)
  - short gastric arteries (from splenic a.) (SS fundus)
  - inferior phrenic arteries
- **Innervation of stomach**
  - ant. + post. vagal trunks
- **Structures that form stomach bed**
  - part of diaphragm
  - L. suprarenal gland
  - U. pole of L. kidney
  - spleen
  - pancreas
  - splenic a.
  - mesentery of transverse colon
- **Transpyloric plane (L1)**
  - midway between jugular notch and pubic symphysis, at tip of ninth costal cartilage, between supracolic and infracolic compartments
  - structures crossed by the plane
  - fundus of gallbladder (RHS)
  - head, neck and body of pancreas
  - left and right hilum of kidneys
  - origin of superior mesenteric a.
  - root of transverse mesocolon
  - duodenojejunal flexure
  - second part of duodenum
  - end of spinal cord
- **Greater omentum**
  - developed from dorsal mesentery
  - double layer of peritoneum
  - from greater curvature of stomach + first part of duodenum → fold back up to enclose transverse colon
- **Lesser omentum**
  - double layer of peritoneum
  - from liver → lesser curvature of stomach + first part of duodenum
- **Lesser sac**
  - space behind stomach (connected to greater sac via epiploic foramen)

- **Epiploic foramen (opening of lesser sac)**
  - post. relationships: IVC
  - ant. relationships: free border of lesser omentum (bile duct + hepatic a. + portal vein)
  - sup. relationships: caudate process of liver
  - inf. relationships: first part of duodenum
- **Retroperitoneal structures**
  - third part of duodenum
  - ascending and descending colon
  - pancreas (except tail)
  - kidney
  - ureter
  - adrenal gland
  - IVC
  - abdominal aorta
  - anal canal
- **Relationships of parts of duodenum**
  - (a) First part of duodenum (superior part)
    - ant: quadrate lobe of liver
    - post: lesser sac, gastroduodenal artery
    - sup: epiploic foramen
    - inf: head of pancreas
  - (b) Second part of duodenum (descending part)
    - ant: fundus of gallbladder, right lobe of liver, transverse colon, small intestine
    - post: hilum of right kidney, right psoas
    - lat: right colic flexure
      med: head of pancreas
  - (c) Third part of duodenum (inferior part) (longest part of duodenum)
    - ant: root of the mesentery
    - post: right ureter
    - sup: head of pancreas
    - inf: jejunum coils
  - (d) Fourth part of duodenum (ascending part)
    - ant: beginning of root of mesentery
    - post: medial border of left psoas
- **Level of umbilicus: L3/4 vertebrae**
- **Linea alba**
  - fibrous line in the middle separating rectus sheaths on either side
  - used in midline incision in surgeries
- **Rectus sheath**
  - encloses rectus abdominis and pyramidalis
  - upper quarter (above mid-point between umbilicus and pubic symphysis)
    - (i) external oblique aponeurosis is anterior to rectus abdominis
    - (ii) internal oblique aponeurosis is split to enclose rectus abdominis
    - (iii) transversus abdominis is behind rectus abdominis

   – lower quarter (below mid-point between umbilicus and pubic symphysis)
         (i) all aponeuroses pass anterior to rectus abdominis
         (ii) rectus abdominis lies in contact with transversus fascia
   – arcuate line (point where inferior epigastric vessels enter rectus sheath)
         (i) midway between umbilicus and pubic symphysis
         (ii) below arcuate line → aponeuroses run ant. to rectus abdominis
- **Useful dermatomes to remember**
  T4 = nipple
  T7 = epigastrium
  T8 = costal margin
  T10 = umbilicus
  T12 = pubic symphysis
  L1 = inguinal ligament
- **Structures on posterior surfaces of liver**
  – abdominal oesophagus
  – stomach (fundus)
  – right colic flexure
  – right kidney
  – diaphragm
  – inferior vena cava (IVC)
- Liver divided into anatomical R. + L. lobes by line drawn from fossa of gallbladder to vena cava
- **Contents of porta hepatis (portal triad)**
  – R. and L. hepatic ducts (bile from liver to c. hepatic duct)
  – R. and L. branches of hepatic artery (branch of coeliac trunk)
  – portal vein
  – sympathetic and parasympathetic fibres
  – hepatic lymph nodes
- **Portal vein**
  = union of splenic vein and superior mesenteric vein at level L2 behind head of pancreas
- **Tributaries of portal vein**
  – splenic vein
  – inf. mesenteric vein (joins splenic vein behind body of pancreas)
  – sup. mesenteric vein (joins splenic vein behind neck of pancreas)
  – R. + L. gastric vein
- **Gallbladder**
  – stores and concentrates bile
  – fundus + body + neck
  – connected to cystic duct → joins c. hepatic duct → CBD
- Arterial SS of gallbladder: cystic artery (branch from R. hepatic a.)
  Venous drainage of gallbladder: cystic vein (drains to portal v.)
- **Biliary tree**
  – R. hepatic duct + L. hepatic duct → common hepatic duct
  – common hepatic duct + cystic duct → common bile duct
- Ligamentum teres = remnant of umbilical vein, found in falciform ligament

- Hepatorenal recess (on RHS) = Morrison's pouch
  Recto-uterine pouch = pouch of Douglas
- **Ampulla of Vater**
  = union of common bile duct (CBD) and main pancreatic duct in second part of duodenum
    - contains smooth muscle sphincter of Oddi regulating flow of bile and pancreatic juice
- **Sites of portocaval anastomoses**
    - lower end of oesophagus (between oesophageal branches of left gastric veins and oesophageal veins draining to azygos vein) → oesophageal varices
    - lower end of GI tract (rectum and anal canal) (between superior rectal vein and middle rectal vein) → haemorrhoids
    - around umbilicus (between para-umbilical veins and left branch of portal vein) → caput medusa
    - retroperitoneal veins
- Dorsal pancreatic bud forms most of the pancreatic head, neck, body and tail
  Ventral pancreatic bud forms inferior head and uncinate process
- **Parts of pancreas**
    - head, neck (level L1), uncinate process, body and tail
- **Relationships of pancreas**
    - ant.: transverse mesocolon + transverse colon, stomach
    - post.: IVC, portal vein, splenic vein, aorta, L. psoas muscle, L. kidney
- **Comparison of jejunum and ileum**
  (*see* Table 4.1)
- **Features of colon**
    - taenia coli (three bands) (from base of appendix → recto-sigmoid junction)
    - haustra
    - appendices epiploicae

Table 4.1 Comparison of jejunum and ileum

Jejunum	Ileum
Proximal two-fifths of small intestine	Distal three-fifths of small intestine
Located in LUQ	Located in RLQ
Larger diameter	Smaller diameter
Thicker wall	Thinner wall
Larger plicae circulares	Smaller plicae circulares
Less prominent arterial arcades	More prominent arterial arcades
Longer vasa recta	Shorter vasa recta
Less mesenteric fat	More mesenteric fat
Does not contain Peyer's patches	Contains Peyer's patches

- **Movements of colon**
  - segmentation (absorption of water)
  - propulsion (movement of bolus)
- **McBurney's point**
  - two-thirds of the distance from the umbilicus to the right anterior superior iliac spine (ASIS)
  - site of pain in appendicitis
- **Various sites where appendix can be found**
  - retrocaecal (most frequent position)
  - pelvic
  - retrocolic
  - pre-ileal
  - post-ileal
  - subcaecal
- **Spleen**
  - anterior to ribs 9–11
  - diaphragmatic surface + visceral surface (where hilus is located)
  - functions:
    - (i) storage of platelets and monocytes
    - (ii) production of antibodies
    - (iii) filtering of red blood cells
  - relationships:
    - (i) inferiorly: L. colic flexure
    - (ii) medially: L. kidney
    - (iii) anteriorly: stomach
    - (iv) posteriorly: diaphragm, L. costodiaphragmatic recess, L. lung
  - connected to stomach by gastrosplenic ligament (contains short gastric a. + L. gastroepiploic a.)
  - connected to kidney by lienorenal ligament
  - arterial SS: splenic a. (from coeliac trunk)
  - venous drainage to splenic v. → portal v.
  - red pulp (site of red blood cell destruction) + white pulp (lymphoid)
- **Peritoneal ligaments associated with spleen**
  - (a) Gastrosplenic ligament:
    - connects greater curvature of stomach to hilum of spleen
    - contains short and left gastroepiploic vessels
  - (b) Splenorenal ligament:
    - connects L. kidney to spleen
    - contains tail of pancreas and splenic vessels
- **Inguinal ligament**
  - thickened lower border of external oblique aponeurosis
  - runs from anterior superior iliac spine (ASIS) to pubic tubercle
  - medially forms lacunar ligament (extends up to pectineal line)
- **Boundaries of the femoral canal (structures pass from abdomen to upper thigh)**
  - anteriorly: inguinal ligament

- medially: lacunar ligament
- laterally: iliopsoas
- posteriorly: pectineus
- **Contents of the femoral canal (lateral to medial)**
  - femoral nerve
  - genitofemoral nerve
  - femoral artery
  - femoral vein
  - femoral ring
- **Boundaries of femoral ring**
  - anteriorly: inguinal ligament
  - medially: lacunar ligament
  - laterally: medial border of femoral vein
  - posteriorly: pectineus
- **Contents of femoral ring**
  - Cloquet's node
  - lymphatics
- **Mid-inguinal point**
  = mid-point of inguinal ligament (halfway between ASIS and pubic tubercle)
- **Boundaries of inguinal triangle**
  (also known as Hesselbach's triangle)
  - lateral: inferior epigastric artery
  - medial: lateral border of rectus abdominis
  - inferior: inguinal ligament
- External inguinal ring: defect in external oblique aponeurosis for passage of spermatic cord or round ligament en route to scrotum or labia major
- Internal inguinal ring: defect in transversalis fascia for passage of spermatic cord from peritoneal cavity
- **Boundaries of inguinal canal**
  - floor: inguinal lig. + lacunar lig.
  - roof: transversus abdominis, lowest fibres of internal oblique muscles
  - ant.: skin, superficial fascia, aponeurosis of external oblique, internal oblique covers lateral third
  - post.: transversalis fascia, conjoint tendon (medial aspect)
- **Contents of inguinal canal**
  - men: spermatic cord
  - women: round ligament of uterus + genital branch of genitofemoral nerve
- **Structures in spermatic cord (10 in total)**
  - vas deferens
  - pampiniform plexus of veins
  - artery to vas deferens
  - vein from vas deferens
  - cremasteric artery and vein
  - testicular artery
  - sympathetic nerve

- genital branch of genitofemoral nerve (SS cremaster muscle)
- testicular lymphatics
- remnants of processus vaginalis
- **Branches of abdominal aorta**
  (*see* Table 4.2)
- **Branches of coeliac trunk**
  - (a) L. gastric a.: passes up to supply lower oesophagus; descends in lesser omentum along lesser curvature of stomach
  - (b) Splenic a.: runs along U. border of pancreas → passes through lienorenal ligament to hilum of spleen
    - short gastric branch: SS fundus of stomach
    - L. gastroepiploic branch: SS great curvature of stomach
  - (c) Hepatic a.: divides into R. + L. hepatic a.
    - enters porta hepatis
    - R. hepatic a. gives off cystic a.
    - gastroduodenal a.: branches into superior pancreaticoduodenal + R. gastroepiploic branches (SS greater curvature of stomach)
    - R. gastric a.: SS lesser curvature of stomach; anastomoses with L. gastric a.
- **Branches of superior mesenteric artery**
  SS caecum, ascending colon, two-thirds of transverse colon
  - inferior pancreaticoduodenal artery
  - middle colic artery
  - R. colic artery

Table 4.2 Branches from abdominal aorta

	Branches	*Vertebral level from which the artery branches*
Three anterior visceral branches	Coeliac trunk	T12
	Superior mesenteric artery	L1
	Inferior mesenteric artery	L3
Three lateral visceral branches	Suprarenal artery	L1
	Renal artery	L1/L2
	Testicular/ovarian artery	L2
Five lateral abdominal wall branches	Inferior phrenic artery	T12/L1
	Four lumbar arteries	L1–4
Three terminal branches	External iliac artery	L4
	Internal iliac artery	L4
	Median sacral artery	L4

- ileocolic artery
- jejunal and ileal arteries
- **Branches of inferior mesenteric artery**
  SS distal transverse colon, descending colon, sigmoid, rectum
  - L. colic artery
  - sigmoid arteries
  - superior rectal artery (anastomoses with middle and inf. rectal arteries)
- **Branches of external iliac artery**
  - inf. epigastric a. (medial)
  - deep circumflex iliac a. (lateral)
- **Branches of internal iliac artery**
  (anterior division)
    - umbilical a.
    - obturator a.
    - inf. vesical a.
    - middle rectal a.
    - internal pudendal a.
    - uterine a.
    - inf. gluteal a.
    - vaginal a.
  (posterior division)
    - iliolumbar a.
    - lat. sacral a.
    - sup. gluteal a.
- **Lumbar plexus**
  formed within psoas major from ventral rami of L1 to L5
  (a) iliohypogastric nerve (L1)
      motor SS to transversus abdominis, internal oblique
    - sensory SS to skin of mons pubis
  (b) ilio-inguinal nerve (L1)
    - sensory SS to skin of groin, scrotum/labium majus, conjoint tendon
  (c) lateral cutaneous nerve of thigh (L2 and 3) passes under inguinal ligament
    - sensory SS to skin of lateral thigh
  (d) genitofemoral nerve (L1 and 2) divides into genital and femoral branches on the anterior surface of psoas
    - genital branch: passes through deep inguinal ring into inguinal canal to supply cremaster muscle or labium majus
    - femoral branch: passes under inguinal ligament to supply skin of thigh
  (e) femoral n. (L2–4)
    - motor SS to muscles in ant. compartment of thigh
    - sensory SS to skin over ant. thigh, medial leg and medial foot
  (f) obturator n. (L2–4)
    - motor SS to muscles in med. compartment of thigh
    - sensory SS to skin over medial thigh
  (g) lumbosacral trunk (L4 and 5)

- **Sacral plexus (lies on piriformis)**
  - formed from ventral rami of L4 and 5, and S1–4
  - (a) superior gluteal n. (L4 and 5, and S1)
    - motor SS to gluteus medius, gluteus minimus and tensor fasciae latae
  - (b) inferior gluteal n. (L5, and S1 and 2)
    - motor SS to gluteus maximus
  - (c) n. to piriformis (S2)
    - motor SS to piriformis
  - (d) n. to obturator internus and superior gemellus (L5, and S1 and 2)
    - motor SS to obturator internus and superior gemellus
  - (e) post. cutaneous n. of thigh (S2 and 3)
    - sensory SS to skin on post. thigh
  - (f) perforating cutaneous n. (S2 and 3)
    - sensory SS over gluteal fold
  - (g) sciatic n. (L4–S3)
    - (i) tibial n.
    - (ii) common fibular n.
  - (h) pudendal n. (S2–4)
    - motor SS to muscles of perineum
    - sensory SS to skin of perineum
- **Rectum**
  - continuous with sigmoid colon at vertebral level S3
  - dilated at lower part (ampulla)
  - U. two-thirds covered by peritoneum ant. and U. third covered by peritoneum lat.
  - puborectalis forms sling at junction between rectum and anal canal, forming anorectal angle
- **Relationships of rectum**
  - ant.: bladder/uterus, prostate and seminal vesicles/vagina
  - post.: sacrum and coccyx
- **Arterial SS of rectum**
  - sup. rectal a. (from inf. mesenteric a.)
  - middle rectal a. (from internal iliac a.)
  - distal part: inf. rectal (from internal pudendal a.)
- **Venous drainage of rectum**
  - proximal part: inf. mesenteric v. → splenic v. → portal v.
  - distal part: iliac v. → IVC

Common pathologies

Causes of oral ulcers
- Dermatological disorders
- Viral infection (herpes simplex)
- Bacterial infection (syphilis)
- Fungal infection (candidiasis)

- Systemic disease (systemic lupus erythematosus)
- Crohn's disease
- Drug induced
- Leukaemia and carcinoma
- Kaposi's sarcoma

Oral cancer
- Squamous-cell carcinoma
- Risk factors: alcohol abuse, smoking
- Symptoms:
  - mass in oral cavity
  - leukoplakia (white patch)
  - ulceration
  - pain when opening mouth
- Signs: cervical lymphadenopathy
- Investigations: biopsy of masses
- Management: surgery, radiotherapy

Parotitis
- Causes: bacterial or viral infection
- Symptoms: painful swelling of parotid gland
- Management: broad-spectrum antibiotics

Achalasia
= inability of the lower oesophageal sphincter to relax during swallowing
- Can predispose to squamous-cell carcinoma of oesophagus
- Symptoms:
  - dysphagia
  - regurgitation and aspiration
  - weight loss
- Investigations:
  - endoscopy
  - barium swallow
  - manometry
  - CXR (dilated oesophagus)
  - CT scan
- Management:
  - forceful dilatation of sphincter
  - surgical myotomy

Pharyngeal pouch
= mucosal protrusion between thyropharyngeus above and cricopharyngeus below
- Formed as a result of increased intraluminal pressure
- Symptoms:
  - dysphagia

- regurgitation
- palpable neck swelling
- Investigations:
  - barium swallow
- Management for symptomatic patients:
  - surgical resection of pouch

Gastro-oesophageal reflux

- Associated with incompetent lower oesophageal sphincter
- Causes:
  - delayed gastric emptying
  - caffeine intake, which relaxes lower oesophageal sphincter
  - hiatus hernia
  - increased intra-abdominal pressure (due to pregnancy or obesity)
  - smoking
- Symptoms:
  - 'heartburn'
  - pain exacerbated by lying down
  - regurgitation
- Complications:
  - Barrett's oesophagus and complicating maligancy (adenocarcinoma)
  - oesophagitis
- Investigations:
  - endoscopy
  - biopsy
  - barium swallow
- Management:
  - smoking cessation
  - antacids
  - proton pump inhibitors (PPIs)
  - H_2-receptor antagnoists
  - weight loss for obese patients

Dyspepsia

- Also known as indigestion
- Causes:
  - oesophageal motility disorders
  - acute gastritis
  - gallstones
  - peptic ulcer
  - drugs (NSAIDs)
  - psychological factors
- Investigations:
  - ultrasound scan of U. abdomen
  - endoscopy
  - test for *Helicobacter pylori*

Oesophagitis
- Presents with chest pain and pain on swallowing
- Most common cause is gastro-oesophageal reflux
- Other causes:
  - consumption of corrosive agents (e.g. bleach)
  - drugs (NSAIDs)
  - infection (candidiasis)
- Can lead to Barrett's oesophagus

Barrett's oesophagus
- Long-standing reflux causes metaplasia of lower oesophagus epithelial cells from stratified squamous to columnar epithelium
- Mostly occurs in lower third of oesophagus
- Hallmark is goblet cells in columnar epithelium
- Complications:
  - oesophageal adenocarcinoma
  - peptic ulcer
- Investigations:
  - endoscopy
  - biopsy

Causes of stricture in oesophagus
- Ingestion of corrosive agents
- Compression caused by tumour of bronchus
- Post-operative scarring after resection of oesophagus
- Gastro-oesophageal reflux
- Oesophageal carcinoma
- Post-radiotherapy
- Functional stricture: achalasia

Oesophageal perforation
- Most commonly due to endoscopic perforation
- May occur after forceful retching or vomiting ('Boerhaave's syndrome')
- Investigations:
  - endoscopy
  - CT scan
- Management: surgery

Oesophageal carcinoma
Squamous-cell carcinoma
- Much more common
- Mostly occurs in middle and lower third of oesophagus
- Risk factors:
  - chronic alcohol intake
  - smoking

- high content of nitrosamines in diet
- coeliac disease
- achalasia

Adenocarcinoma
- Mostly occurs in lower third of oesophagus
- Risk factors:
  - Barrett's oesophagus
  - long-standing gastro-oesophageal reflux disease
- Symptoms:
  - dysphagia (typically progressive and painless)
  - regurgitation and aspiration
  - weight loss
  - anaemia
- U. oesophageal tumour may invade L. recurrent laryngeal nerve →
  hoarseness of voice
- Investigations:
  - CXR (staging)
  - endoscopy and biopsy
  - barium swallow (filling defect)
  - thoracic and abdominal CT scans (staging)
- Management: surgical removal and radiotherapy

Acute gastritis
= inflammation of stomach
- Self-limiting condition
- Common causes:
  - alcohol
  - drugs (especially NSAIDs)
  - ingestion of corrosive agents
  - bile reflux
  - *H. pylori* infection
  - viral infection (especially cytomegalovirus)
  - physiological stress (e.g. burns)

Chronic gastritis
- Causes:
  - autoimmune reaction to parietal cells (pernicious anaemia)
  - chronic *H. pylori* infection
  - alcohol
- Autoimmune gastritis: patients have auto-Ab against intrinsic factor or
  gastric parietal cells, leading to destruction of related gland cells that results
  in loss of acid secretion (achlorhydria) and pernicious anaemia (loss of
  intrinsic factor)
- *H. pylori*-associated gastritis: treated by antibiotic treatment; mostly involves
  antrum; associated with increased risk of developing gastric ulcer

Peptic ulceration
- Most common in oesophagus, first part of duodenum and stomach
- Mostly occurs in *H. pylori*-infected patients
- Other causes:
  - use of NSAIDs
  - Zollinger–Ellison syndrome (non-insulin-secreting tumour of pancreas produces gastrin-like hormone)
  - severe burns (Curling's ulcer)
- Symptoms:
  - recurrent epigastric pain, typically 2 hours after a meal, relieved by intake of milk
- Signs:
  - dyspepsia
  - rigid abdomen (if perforation occurs)
- Investigations:
  - endoscopy
- Complications:
  - haemorrhage
  - perforation
  - obstruction
  - anaemia
  - malignancy
- Presence of *H. pylori* is confirmed by urease test (*H. pylori* splits urea to release ammonia)
- *H. pylori* is eradicated by proton pump inhibitors (e.g. omeprazole) and antimicrobial drugs (clarithromycin and metronidazole)
- Management:
  - stop use of NSAIDs
  - give antacids
- Perforated peptic ulcer (PPU) = severe pain of sudden onset aggravated by movement; CXR usually shows free gas under diaphragm

Gastric cancer
- Mostly adenocarcinomas
- Risk factors:
  - age 70 years or older
  - male sex
  - high content of pickled and salted food in diet
  - smoking
  - alcohol abuse
  - *H. pylori* infection
  - chronic gastritis
  - family history of gastric cancer
  - blood group A
  - hereditary non-polyposis colorectal cancer syndrome (HNPCC)
  - hypertrophic gastropathy

- Mostly occurs in pylorus and antrum
- Two types: intestinal and diffuse (Lauren classification)
  - (a) Intestinal type: exophytic growth; microscopically shows mucin-producing cells
  - (b) Diffuse type: ulcerative or diffuse infiltrative growth (linitis plastica, also known as leather-bottle stomach); microscopically shows mucin-producing signet-ring cells
- If spreads to left supraclavicular nodes = Virchow's node (Troisier's sign)
- If spreads to periumbilical lymph nodes = Sister Mary Joseph's sign
- If spreads to ovaries = Krukenberg tumour
- Symptoms:
  - nausea
  - vomiting
  - persistent epigastric pain or discomfort
  - dyspepsia
  - unexplained weight loss
  - anorexia
  - dysphagia
  - haematemesis
  - change in bowel habits
- Signs:
  - iron-deficiency anaemia
  - melaena
  - epigastric mass
  - Virchow's node
- Investigations:
  - full blood count
  - barium meal
  - gastroscopy
  - biopsy
  - CT scan (staging)
- Management:
  - surgical resection
  - chemotherapy

Complications of gastrectomy
- Weight loss
- Bile reflux gastritis
- Dumping (rapid gastric emptying → hyperosmotic contents in small intestine draw water to lumen → abdominal discomfort after eating)
- Diarrhoea
- Iron-deficiency anaemia and pernicious anaemia (caused by vitamin B_{12} deficiency)

Gastrointestinal stromal tumour (GIST)
- Tumour arising from interstitial cells of Cajal

- Mutations in c-Kit
- Investigations: endoscopy and biopsy

Hiatal hernia
- Two types, usually occurring in stomach

Sliding hiatus hernia
- Represents 90% of hiatus hernias
- Herniation of abdominal organ through oesophageal hiatus in diaphragm
- Gastroesophageal junction displaced above diaphragm (acid-secreting parts of stomach above diaphragmatic constriction)
- Risk factors:
  - obesity
  - ageing
- Symptoms:
  - heartburn due to gastro-oesophageal reflux
  - relieved by antacids
- Investigations:
  - barium swallow
  - 24-hour oesophageal pH monitoring
- Management:
  - elevation of head of bed
  - avoid intake of coffee
  - give H_2-antagonists (e.g. ranitidine)
  - give proton pump inhibitors
  - surgery (if complications occur)
- Complications:
  - oesophagitis
  - oesophageal stricture
  - ulceration
  - adenocarcinoma

Rolling hiatus hernia
- Represents 10% of hiatus hernias
- Herniation due to abdominal organ pushing up beside oesophagus
- Gastroesophageal junction remains below diaphragm
- Herniated part of stomach may strangulate and infarct
- Symptoms:
  - chest pain
  - dysphagia due to oesophageal compression
- Ligament of Treitz
  = anatomical landmark for the duodeno-jejunal junction
  - connects duodenum to diaphragm

Jaundice
- Investigations:
  - ultrasound (dilated bile ducts)

  – liver function tests

Pre-hepatic jaundice
- Caused by increased breakdown of red blood cells
- Increased production of bilirubin
- Haemolytic anaemia

Hepatic jaundice
- Caused by inflammation of liver
- Liver cirrhosis, drug-induced damage and hepatitis
- Increased unconjugated and conjugated bilirubin

Post-hepatic jaundice
- Extrahepatic causes:
  – gallstones in CBD (most common)
  – tumour at head of pancreas
  – pancreatitis
  – cholangiocarcinoma
- Intrahepatic causes:
  – drug induced
  – alcohol
  – bacterial infection
  – primary sclerosing cholangitis
  – autoimmune hepatitis
  – pregnancy
- Symptoms:
  – pruritus
  – dark urine and pale stools
  – jaundice
  – steatorrhoea and weight loss (due to malabsorption)

Courvoisier's law
Obstructive jaundice occurs when there is a palpable gallbladder that is not due to gallstones (because gallstones would result in a small contracted gallbladder)

Gilbert's syndrome
- Congenital condition
- Reduction in activity of glucuronyl transferase
- Non-haemolytic hyperbilirubinaemia
- Causes pre-hepatic jaundice

Causes of hepatomegaly
- Heart failure
- Liver cancer (metastatic is more common than primary)
- Cirrhosis
- Hepatitis
- Polycystic liver
- Leukaemia

- Liver abscess
- Amyloidosis
- Glycogen storage disease

Acute hepatitis
- Risk factors:
  - alcohol
  - viral infections
  - drugs
- Symptoms include acute jaundice and malaise

Viral hepatitis
Hepatitis A
- Sources:
  - shellfish
  - unhygienic water sources
- Faecal–oral transmission
- Diagnostic feature: anti-HAV IgM
- No carrier state

Hepatitis B
- Transmission routes:
  - vertical (mother to child)
  - sharing of needles
  - infected blood products
  - sexual
- Diagnostic features:
  - HBsAg, HBeAg
  - anti-HBc
- Investigations:
  - PCR
  - viral load in blood and HBV DNA
- Management:
  - treat chronic hepatitis to avoid cirrhosis/hepatoma
  - interferon
  - adefovir (nephrotoxic)
  - lamivudine

Hepatitis C
- Transmission routes:
  - IV drug misuse
  - vertical (mother to child)
  - blood transfusion
- Diagnostic feature: hepatitic C RNA
- Management:
  - treatment with IFN and ribavirin

Hepatitis D
- Occurs simultaneously as hepatitis B infection; superimpose on hepatitis B infection
- Diagnostic feature: anti-HDV IgM

Hepatitis E
- Faecal–oral transmission
- Diagnostic feature: anti-HEV IgM

Chronic hepatitis (> 6 months)
- Causes:
  - alcohol
  - chronic viral hepatitis
  - haemochromatosis (iron overload causing browning of skin)
  - autoimmune liver disease
  - steatohepatitis
  - α_1-antitrypsin deficiency (liver damage and emphysema)
  - Wilson's disease
- Complications:
  - liver failure
  - hepatocellular carcinoma
  - cirrhosis

Wilson's disease
- Autosomal recessive
- Disorder of copper metabolism
- Copper accumulates in liver and brain
- Symptoms:
  - Kayser–Fleischer rings in cornea
- Investigations:
  - blood tests (reduced serum copper and caeruloplasmin levels)
  - urinary copper levels (raised)
  - liver biopsy
- Management:
  - penicillamine (chelates copper)

Budd–Chiari syndrome
= blockage of venous outflow of liver due to obstruction of hepatic vein
- Causes:
  - idiopathic
  - oral contraceptive pill
  - polycythaemia vera
  - hepatic infection
  - liver trauma
- Investigations:
  - ultrasound

- CT scan
- Management:
  - thrombolytic therapy
  - transjugular intrahepatic portosystemic shunt (TIPS)
  - liver transplant

Liver abscess

Pyogenic abscess
- Usually caused by ascending infection from cholangitis
- Symptoms:
  - RUQ pain
  - fever
  - jaundice
  - vomiting
  - rigors
- Signs: hepatomegaly
- Investigations:
  - blood tests (raised serum ALP)
  - CXR (elevation of hemidiaphragm)
  - ultrasound
  - CT scan
- Management:
  - aspiration of abscess
  - antibiotics

Amoebic abscess
- Usually caused by *Entamoeba histolytica*
- Symptoms:
  - malaise
  - anorexia
  - abdominal pain
  - fever
  - diarrhoea
- Complications:
  - rupture of abscess
  - septicaemia
- Investigations:
  - aspiration of cyst
  - ELISA test for amoeba
- Management:
  - metronidazole
  - aspiration of abscess

Autoimmune liver disease
There are two forms.

Autoimmune hepatitis
- Anti-smooth-muscle Ab in bloodstream
- Anti-nuclear Ab in bloodstream
- Symptoms:
  - anorexia
  - jaundice
  - malaise
- Association with other coexisting autoimmune diseases (e.g. pernicious anaemia)
- Management: corticosteroids

Primary biliary cirrhosis
- Anti-mitochondrial Ab (AMA) in bloodstream in over 95% of patients
- Symptoms:
  - pruritus
  - arthralgia
  - lethargy
- Signs:
  - weight loss
  - hepatomegaly
  - jaundice
- Investigations:
  - LFT (ALP) → high ALP is often the only abnormality
  - blood tests (increased AMA, IgM and cholesterol levels)
  - liver biopsy
  - ultrasound
- Complications:
  - liver cirrhosis

Steatohepatitis
= fatty liver and inflammation
- Alcoholic steatohepatitis, caused by alcohol, is the most common type
- Non-alcoholic steatohepatitis is associated with metabolic syndrome (diabetes, obesity and dyslipidaemia)

Alcoholic liver disease
- Causes fatty liver and chronic hepatitis
- Characteristic histological features:
  - Mallory's hyaline
  - central hyaline sclerosis
  - neutrophil infiltration
  - liver cirrhosis
- Signs:
  - palmar erythema
  - Dupuytren's contracture
  - jaundice

- hepatomegaly
- ascites
- Investigations:
  - history taking
  - GGT in blood

Liver cirrhosis
= chronic liver cell death with nodular regeneration and fibrosis
- Classified on the basis of size of regenerative nodules into micronodular or macronodular, or by aetiology (alcoholic, viral, biliary or autoimmune)
- Causes:
  - chronic hepatitis B or C viral infection
  - alcohol abuse
  - non-alcoholic steatohepatitis (NASH)
  - autoimmune liver disease, including primary biliary cirrhosis
  - idiopathic causes
  - α_1-antitrypsin deficiency
  - Wilson's disease
  - haemochromatosis
  - non-alcoholic fatty liver disease (NAFLD)
  - glycogen storage disease
- Signs:
  - jaundice
  - finger clubbing
  - Dupuytren's contracture
  - palmar erythema
  - hepatic flap
  - spider naevi on chest
  - purpura
  - loss of axillary hair
  - ascites
  - hepatomegaly
  - splenomegaly
- Complications:
  - liver failure
  - portal hypertension
  - hepatocellular carcinoma
  - portal vein thrombosis
  - hepatic encephalopathy
  - hepato-renal syndrome
- Investigations:
  - FBC
  - LFT
  - ultrasound scan of liver
  - liver biopsy
  - CT scan

- MRI scan
- endoscopy (for varices)
- Prognosis determined by Child–Pugh score

Acute liver failure
- Causes:
  - excessive alcohol intake
  - drug induced
  - fulminant viral hepatitis
  - decompensated cirrhosis
  - Wilson's disease
  - heart failure
  - shock
  - metastases
- Symptoms:
  - malaise and altered sensorium
  - jaundice
  - nausea
  - vomiting
  - hepatic encephalopathy
- Signs:
  - jaundice
  - hepatic flap
  - ascites
- Investigations:
  - prothrombin time (increased), serum albumin concentration (decreased)
  - blood tests for virus markers
  - serum copper levels
  - IgM anti-HBc
  - ultrasound scan of liver
- Complications:
  - infection
  - hypoglycaemia
  - hepato-renal failure
  - hepatic encephalopathy
  - metabolic acidosis
- Management: transplantation

Chronic liver failure
= inability of liver to perform normal physiological functions
- Mostly caused by liver cirrhosis
- Clinical features (due to chronic hepatocellular dysfunction or portal hypertension):
  - jaundice
  - ascites
  - variceal bleeding (due to portal hypetension)

- peripheral oedema
- Investigations:
  - prothrombin time (prolonged)
  - bilirubin level (increased)
  - albumin level in blood (low)

Portal hypertension
- Most common cause: cirrhosis
- Other causes (according to sites of obstruction):
  - (a) extrahepatic pre-sinusoid:
    - portal vein thrombosis
  - (b) intrahepatic pre-sinusoid:
    - schistosomiasis
    - granulomata
  - (c) sinusoid:
    - liver cirrhosis
    - metastatic liver disease
    - congenital hepatic fibrosis
  - (d) intrahepatic post-sinusoid:
    - veno-occlusive disease
  - (e) extrahepatic post-sinusoid:
    - Budd–Chiari syndrome
- Symptoms:
  - haematemesis
  - melaena
  - haematochezia
- Signs:
  - splenomegaly
- Complications:
  - oesophageal varices
  - ascites
  - hepatic encephalopathy
- Investigations:
  - endoscopy
  - ultrasound scan of spleen
- Management:
  - endoscopic sclerotherapy
  - band ligation
  - transjugular intrahepatic portosystemic shunt (TIPS)

Ascites
= presence of fluid in peritoneal cavity
- Causes of transudate:
  - liver cirrhosis
  - heart failure
  - Budd–Chiari syndrome

- Causes of exudate:
  - peritonitis
  - pancreatitis
  - nephrotic syndrome
- Investigations:
  - aspiration of fluid (cytology, culture and Gram stain for bacteria)
- Management:
  - paracentesis
  - diuretics (spironolactone)

Benign liver tumours
- Haemangioma (most common type)
- Hepatic adenoma
- Focal nodular hyperplasia (FNH)

Hepatocellular carcinoma (HCC) (liver cancer)
- Risk factors:
  - cirrhosis
  - portal hypertension
  - carriers of hepatitis B or C
  - alcohol abuse
  - haemochromatosis
  - aflatoxin
- Symptoms:
  - fever
  - painful hepatomegaly (presents late)
  - abdominal mass
  - anorexia
  - weight loss
  - jaundice
  - ascites
  - RUQ pain
  - splenomegaly
- Investigations:
  - blood tests (tumour marker α-fetoprotein, AFP)
  - ultrasound scan
  - liver biopsy
  - CT scan with IV contrast
- Management:
  - hepatic resection
  - radiofrequency ablation (RFA)
  - chemo-embolisation
  - liver transplant

Biliary diseases

Cholelithiasis

= presence of gallstones in the gallbladder

- Composition of stones:
  - mixed (most common)
  - cholesterol
  - pigment
  - calcium carbonate
- Causes biliary colic: transient obstruction of cystic duct results in recurrent sudden pain in abdominal area, which tends to be more severe after meals
- Risk factors – 5F's:
  - female
  - forty
  - fat
  - flatulent
  - fertile
- Symptoms:
  - postprandial abdominal pain
  - nausea
  - vomiting
- Signs:
  - RUQ tenderness
- Investigations:
  - ultrasound scan
  - endoscopic retrograde cholangiopancreatography (ERCP)
  - percutaneous cholangiography
  - CT scan
- Management:
  - pain relief
  - oral bile acid (ursodeoxycholic acid)
  - cholecystectomy
  - lithotripsy
- Complications:
  - mucocoele
  - biliary pancreatitis
  - acute cholangitis
  - acute cholecystitis
  - formation of biliary enteric fistula
  - choledocholithiasis
  - gallbladder empyema
  - porcelain gallbladder
  - gallbladder cancer

Acute cholecystitis

= acute inflammation of gallbladder, most commonly caused by stone impaction in cystic duct, obstructing bile outflow

- Symptoms:
  - fever
  - severe pain (mimics biliary colic, but lasts longer and is often associated with rebound tenderness)
  - anorexia
- Signs:
  - Murphy's sign (inspiratory arrest during deep palpation of RUQ)
- Investigations:
  - blood tests (increased WCC)
  - ultrasound scan (gallstones)
  - physical examination
- Complications:
  - empyema of gallbladder
  - gangrene of gallbladder
  - gallstone ileus
- Management:
  - analgesics
  - IV fluid administration
  - antibiotics
  - cholecystectomy

Choledocholithiasis

= presence of gallstones in common bile duct (CBD), which can result in stasis of bile in liver, causing cholangitis
- Symptoms:
  - RUQ pain
  - jaundice
  - fever
  - biliary colic
- Characteristic feature:
  - marked increase in alkaline phosphatase (ALP) activity
- Complications:
  - acute pancreatitis
  - ascending cholangitis
- Investigations:
  - ultrasound scan
  - ERCP
- Management:
  - ERCP to remove bile duct stones

Cholangitis

= inflammation of biliary tract
- Common cause: gallstone blocking common bile duct (choledocholithiasis)
- Common organisms involved: Gram-negative organisms (*E. coli*, *Klebsiella*), *Enterococcus*
- Can lead to septic shock if not detected early
- Symptoms (Charcot's triad): fever, RUQ pain and jaundice

- Investigations:
  - blood tests (increased WCC)
  - ultrasound scan
- Management:
  - decompression of biliary tree
  - IV fluid administration
  - urgent ERCP

Cholangiocarcinoma

= bile duct cancer
- Mostly adenocarcinomas
- Can be intra- or extra-hepatic ducts
- Common presentation:
  - painless obstructive jaundice
  - fatigue
  - pruritus
  - weight loss
  - RUQ pain
- Signs:
  - jaundice
  - dark urine
  - pale-coloured stools
- Investigations:
  - ERCP
- Management:
  - palliative stenting

Klatskin's tumour

= cholangiocarcinoma of bile duct at junction of R. and L. hepatic ducts

Gallbladder cancer

- Most commonly adenocarcinoma
- Associated with cholelithiasis and porcelain gallbladder
- Symptoms:
  - RUQ pain
  - anorexia
  - jaundice
  - weight loss
- Management: cholecystectomy

Upper GI bleeding

- Mostly caused by duodenal ulcers
- Other possible causes:
  - oesophageal varices
  - gastric ulcers
- Risk factors:
  - long-standing vomiting

- trauma
- large alcohol intake
- smoking
- anticoagulation therapy
- use of NSAIDs

Haematemesis
= vomiting of bright red blood/coffee-ground emesis

Melaena
= black, tarry stools seen in patients with bleeding of upper GI tract

Lower GI bleeding
- Bleeding per rectum
- Common causes:
  - haemorrhoids
  - diverticular disease
  - anal fissure (if associated with painful bowel movement)

Haematochezia
= bright red blood from rectum

Meckel's diverticulum
- Congenital disease
- Remnant of vitelline duct of embryo (connects yolk sac to midgut)
- Rule of twos: occurs in 2% of population, 2 feet from ileo-caecal valve, mostly 2 inches long
- Most patients are asymptomatic (2% are symptomatic), and the main complaint is of painless rectal bleeding
- Mostly incidental findings
- Complications:
  - bleeding
  - intestinal obstruction
  - formation of fistula
- Management:
  - surgical resection (if bleeding or obstruction occurs)

Coeliac disease
- Inflammatory disorder of small bowel
- Most commonly affects proximal small bowel
- Can cause malabsorption
- Symptoms:
  (a) infants:
    - failure to thrive
  (b) children:

- stunted growth
(c) adults:
  - iron-deficiency anaemia
  - mouth ulcers
  - steatorrhoea
  - bloating
  - anaemia
  - weight loss
  - malaise
- Investigations:
  - endoscopy and biopsy of small bowel
  - blood tests (antibodies)
- Complications:
  - increased risk of colon cancer
- Management:
  - gluten-free diet

Inflammatory bowel disease (IBD)

Table 4.3 Comparison of Crohn's disease and ulcerative colitis

Features	Crohn's disease	Ulcerative colitis
Involvement	Segmental (skip lesions) From mouth to anus, mostly in terminal ileum and colon	Continuous from rectum backward for variable distance Large intestine only
Layers affected	Transmural	Mucosal only
Granulomas	Non-caseating granulomas	None
Wall appearance	Thickened with formation of strictures; creeping fat	Thinned with dilated lumen; crypt abscesses
Mucosal changes	'Cobblestone' appearance	Superficial ulceration with pseudopolyps
Fissures and fistulae	Yes	No
Increase in cancer risk	5- to 6-fold	20- to 30-fold
Presence of pseudopolyps	No	Yes (between ulcers)
Barium enema findings	String sign (strictures), cobblestone mucosa	Lead pipe appearance (loss of haustrations due to oedema)
Surgery	Only in cases of small bowel obstruction (conservative management is indicated)	Yes, if uncontrolled (removal of colon and rectum with ileostomy)

- Signs of Crohn's disease:
  - abdominal pain
  - diarrhoea

- anaemia
- fever
- malaise
- weight loss
- positive occult blood
- extra-intestinal manifestations (uveitis, erythema nodosum)
- Signs of ulcerative colitis:
  - anaemia
  - bloody diarrhoea with mucus
  - fever
  - abdominal pain
  - weight loss
  - malaise
  - extra-intestinal manifestations (iritis, uveitis, ankylosing spondylitis, primary sclerosing cholangitis, erythema nodosum)
- Investigations:
  - AXR
  - rectal examination (ulcerative colitis)
  - sigmoidoscopy
  - proctoscopy
  - colonoscopy and biopsy
  - barium enema
  - high-resolution ultrasound scan
- Complications:
  - local: toxic megacolon, increased risk of malignancy, haemorrhage, perforation, fistula formation, obstruction
  - general: weight loss, anaemia
- Management:
  - infliximab (Crohn's disease)
  - IV corticosteroids (ulcerative colitis)
  - proctocolectomy

Small bowel obstruction (SBO)
- Common causes:
  - post-operative adhesions
  - hernia
  - foreign bodies
  - neoplasms
  - gallstone ileus
  - volvulus
  - intussusception
  - Crohn's disease
  - annular pancreas
  - intramural haematoma
- Symptoms:
  - nausea and vomiting

- decreased or absent stool and flatus
- abdominal pain and discomfort
- abdominal distension
- Signs:
  - high-pitched bowel sounds
- Complications:
  - small bowel strangulation due to closed loop obstruction (present with fever, shock and peritoneal signs)
  - septicaemia
- Investigations:
  - CT with contrast
  - AXR (dilated loops of bowel with air–fluid levels)
- Management:
  - NPO
  - IV fluid resuscitation
  - insert nasogastric tube
  - administer IV fluid
  - insert Foley catheter

Small intestine tumours
- Risk factors:
  - autoimmune disorders
  - Peutz–Jeghers syndrome
  - Crohn's disease

Benign tumours
- Leiomyoma
- Adenoma
- Lipoma
- Hamartoma

Malignant tumours (primary or secondary)
- Primary:
  - adenocarcinoma
  - lymphoma
  - carcinoid
  - sarcoma
- Symptoms:
  - obstruction
  - bleeding
  - diarrhoea
  - abdominal pain
  - weight loss
- Signs:
  - palpable abdominal mass
- Investigations:
  - ultrasound scan

– CT scan

Carcinoid tumour
- Most commonly found in appendix
- Can arise from thymus or other parts of small bowel
- Composed of neuroendocrine cells
- Mostly secrete serotonin, i.e. 5-hydroxytryptamine (5-HT)
- Symptoms (carcinoid syndrome):
  – flushing
  – diarrhoea
  – vomiting
  – abdominal pain
  – bronchospasm
- Investigations:
  – urinary concentration of 5-hydroxyindoleacetic acid (5-HIAA)
  – blood concentration of serotonin
  – barium enema
- Management: surgical resection/targeted radiotherapy for advanced disease

Acute appendicitis
- Caused by obstruction of appendix by faecolith or foreign bodies
- Blood supply to appendix consists of end arteries (from ileocolic artery) → if appendicular arteries become thrombosed → gangrene → risk of perforation → peritonitis/local abscess
- Symptoms:
  – facial flushing
  – fever
  – tenderness in periumbilical region (referred pain) before localising to RLQ (peritoneal irritation)
  – nausea
  – vomiting
  – anorexia
- Signs:
  – tachycardia
  – guarding and rebound tenderness over site of appendicitis
- Complications:
  – perforation
  – peritonitis
  – spread to liver
- Investigations:
  – CBC
  – ultrasound scan
  – AXR
- Management: appendicectomy (grid-iron incision)

Sigmoid volvulus
- Caused by long-standing constipation
- Symptoms:
  - distended abdomen
  - abdominal pain
  - anorexia
  - nausea
  - vomiting
- Investigations:
  - AXR (coffee-bean sign)
  - sigmoidoscopy
  - barium enema
- Management:
  - flexible sigmoidoscopy decompression
  - Hartmann's procedure if strangulation occurs

Large bowel obstruction (LBO)
- Films show dilated bowel with air–fluid levels
- Less fluid and electrolyte disturbance than in SBO
- Common causes:
  - cancer
  - diverticulitis
- Symptoms:
  - marked abdominal distention
  - constipation
- Signs:
  - high-pitched bowel sounds
- Investigations:
  - AXR
  - barium enema
  - CT (staging)
- Management:
  - correct fluid and electrolyte imbalance
  - surgery

Diverticulosis
= outpouchings of GI tract in colon
- Most common site is sigmoid colon, descending colon
- Weakness in bowel wall leads to herniation of mucosa and submucosa through muscular layer of membrane (points of entry of blood supply to colon)
- Risk factors: deficiency of fibre in diet → constipation → sigmoid colon X becomes distended → intraluminal pressure is increased, and long-standing constipation occurs
- Symptoms:
  - suprapubic pain

- constipation
- Signs:
  - local guarding and rigidity
- Investigations:
  - barium enema
- Most common complication:
  - diverticulitis
- Management:
  - encourage the patient to switch to a high-fibre diet

Diverticulitis
= infection and/or perforation of diverticulum
- Symptoms:
  - acute: nausea and vomiting, fever, LLQ pain and guarding
  - chronic: large bowel obstruction, change in bowel habit, PR bleeding and mucus production
- Complications:
  - formation of adhesions
  - perforation (leading to peritonitis, fistula formation and/or pericolic abscess)
  - rectal haemorrhage
  - intestinal obstruction
- Investigations:
  - blood tests (increased WCC)
  - sigmoidoscopy
  - colonoscopy
  - abdominal CT
- Management:
  - broad-spectrum antibiotics and IV fluid replacement
  - drain abscesses percutaneously, and resect fistula
  - perform Hartmann's procedure in acute cases

Angiodysplasia
- Tiny vascular malformations in colon wall
- Most commonly occurs in caecum and ascending colon
- Symptoms:
  - rectal bleeding/haemorrhage
  - iron-deficiency anaemia
- Investigations:
  - angiography
  - colonoscopy (submucosal lesions)
- Management:
  - blood transfusion for severe cases
  - some cases may require R. hemicolectomy

Peutz–Jeghers syndrome
- Autosomal dominant disorder
- Affects small intestine and colon
- Multiple hamartomatous polyps
- Increased risk of colon cancer
- Symptoms:
  - anaemia
  - intussusception
  - pigmentation around lips
- Investigations:
  - colonoscopy

Familial adenomatous polyposis (FAP)
- Autosomal dominant disorder
- Mutation of APC gene (adenomatous polyposis gene) of chromosome 5
- Symptoms:
  - rectal bleeding
- Characteristic lesion:
  - hypertrophy of retinal pigment epithelium (fundoscopy finding)
- Investigations:
  - genetic tests
- Management:
  - proctocolectomy and ileo-anal pouch

Hereditary non-polyposis colorectal cancer (HNPCC)
- Autosomal dominant
- Early age of onset
- Mostly develops in the R. colon
- Adenocarcinoma
- Management: subtotal colectomy

Colorectal cancer
- Sites of incidence (in decreasing order of frequency):
  - rectum
  - sigmoid colon
  - caecum and ascending colon
  - transverse colon
  - descending colon
- Dietary risk factors:
  - low fibre content
  - high intake of red meat
  - high intake of saturated fat
  - low intake of micronutrients (vitamins)
- Other risk factors:
  - age > 50 years

- – familial adenomatous polyposis (FAP)
- – hereditary non-polyposis colorectal cancer (HNPCC)
- – ulcerative colitis
- Symptoms:
  - – change in bowel habits
  - – bleeding
  - – tenesmus

(a) tumours on R. side of colon:
- – mostly ulcerating masses
- – anaemia
- – melaena
- – anorexia
- – loss of weight
- – fatigue

(b) tumours on L. side of colon:
- – 'apple-core' lesion detected by barium enema
- – change in bowel habits (stools of smaller sizes)
- – intestinal obstruction
- – haematochezia
- – anorexia
- – loss of weight

- Metastasis:
  - – haematogenous spread (liver, lungs, bone and brain)
  - – lymphatic spread
  - – local spread
  - – transcoelomic spread
- Dukes' staging:
  - – A: tumour confined to submucosa (survival > 90%)
  - – B: tumour involving muscularis propria (survival $c.$ 70%)
  - – C: tumour involving regional lymph nodes (survival > 30%)
  - – D: distant metastasis
- Investigations:
  - – blood tests (faecal occult blood test, FOBT) (serum CEA)
  - – PR examination (mass and occult blood)
  - – double-contrast barium enema (stricture/filling defect)
  - – rigid sigmoidoscopy
  - – flexible sigmoidoscopy
  - – colonoscopy (biopsy)
  - – abdominal CT (staging)
  - – PET scan (staging)
- Management: R./L. hemicolectomy and adjuvant chemotherapy

Acute pancreatitis
- Risk factors:
  - – gallstones (obstruct pancreatic ducts)
  - – alcohol abuse

- – shock
- – mumps virus
- – Coxsackie virus
- – drugs (corticosteroids)
- – idiopathic
- – trauma
- – iatrogenic (post-ERCP)
- • Symptoms:
  - – severe epigastric pain, mostly radiating to the back
  - – nausea and vomiting
- • Signs:
  - – fever
  - – tachycardia
  - – abdominal tenderness
  - – epigastric tenderness
  - – decreased bowel sounds
  - – dehydration (severe hypovolaemia)
  - – Grey–Turner's sign (in severe cases) = local bruising of skin around flanks due to extravasation of blood from pancreatic haemorrhage
  - – Cullen sign = peri-umbilical bruising
- • Investigations:
  - – blood tests (serum amylase and lipase)
  - – urinary amylase
  - – AXR
  - – ultrasound scan
  - – CT scan with contrast
  - – MRCP
- • Important diagnostic features:
  - – raised blood level of amylase
  - – abdominal X-ray may show sentinel loop sign in upper abdomen
- • Complications:
  - – pseudocyst (most common)
  - – shock
  - – haemorrhage (due to erosion of arteries by released enzymes)
  - – pancreatic necrosis
  - – abscess formation
  - – hyperglycaemia
  - – duodenal obstruction (due to compression by pancreas mass)
  - – fluid and electrolyte imbalance
- • Management:
  - – IV fluids
  - – nasogastric aspiration
  - – analgesia
- • Prognosis determined by Glasgow criteria

Chronic pancreatitis
- Destruction of parenchyma occurs
- Causes:
  - chronic alcohol abuse (most common)
  - autoimmune disease
  - trauma
  - cystic fibrosis
- Symptoms:
  - recurrent epigastric pain radiating to the back between the shoulder blades
  - steatorrhoea
  - weight loss
- Complications:
  - extrahepatic obstructive jaundice due to stricture of CBD by pancreas
  - malabsorption due to loss of exocrine secretions, or diabetes due to loss of endocrine secretions
  - insulin-dependent diabetes mellitus; malnutrition
  - pancreatic pseudocyst
- Investigations:
  - serum amylase levels
  - AXR
  - ultrasound scan
  - MRCP
  - CT (calcifications and pseudocysts)
  - MRI
- Management:
  - dietary fat restriction (for steatorrhoea)
  - replace pancreatic enzymes
  - give narcotics (for pain relief)
  - surgical resection (pancreatico-jejunostomy)

Annular pancreas
- Pancreas completely encircles duodenum, resulting in obstruction
- Management: duodenoduodenostomy bypass

Pancreatic cancer
- Highly malignant
- Most commonly adenocarcinoma from duct cells, mostly in exocrine pancreas
- Most commonly occurs in head of pancreas (present earlier with biliary obstruction)
- Peri-ampullary cancer includes cancer of ampulla, lower bile duct and pancreatic head
- Risk factors:
  - age
  - alcohol abuse

- smoking
- diabetes
- toxins
- Symptoms:
  - epigastric pain
  - painless and progressive obstructive jaundice (in patients with cancer of pancreatic head)
  - back pain
  - weight loss
  - dark urine and pale stool (in patients with cancer of pancreatic head)
  - steatorrhoea
- Signs:
  - cachexia
  - jaundice
  - palpable non-tender GB (Courvoisier's sign in some patients with cancer of pancreatic head)
  - hepatomegaly
  - palpable mass in pancreatic region
- Investigations:
  - blood tests, tumour markers (CEA, CA 19–9)
  - ultrasound scan
  - abdominal CT
  - ERCP
- Very poor prognosis because it presents late
- Management: Whipple procedure = pancreatico-duodenectomy (for cancer of head of pancreas)

Neuroendocrine tumours of pancreas
- Types:
  - insulinoma (mostly benign)
  - gastrinoma (secretes gastric acid)
  - glucagonoma (alpha-cell tumour)
  - somatostatinoma (D-cell tumour)

Causes of splenomegaly
- Congestive heart failure
- Bacterial infection (TB)
- Viral infection (Epstein–Barr)
- Cirrhosis
- Portal hypertension
- Portal vein thrombosis
- Thalassaemia
- Megaloblastic anaemia
- Chronic myeloid leukaemia (CML)
- SLE
- Sarcoidosis

- Amyloidosis
- Lymphoma

Peritonitis
= inflammation of peritoneal cavity
- Causes:
    - rupture of intra-abdominal abscess
    - transmural spread
    - perforation of small bowel
- Signs:
    (a) localised peritonitis:
        - guarding
        - rebound tenderness
    (b) generalised peritonitis:
        - rigid abdomen
        - absent bowel sounds
        - may cause paralytic ileus
- Investigations:
    - CXR (free gas under diaphragm)
    - ultrasound scan
    - CT scan

Perianal abscesses
- Types:
    - pelvirectal
    - ischiorectal
    - submucous
    - perianal
- Causes:
    - infection of glands
- Symptoms:
    - pain in anal region
- Management:
    - give antibiotics
    - drain abscess

Haemorrhoids
= congested vascular cushions around lower rectum and/or anus, caused by varicose veins
- Mostly occur at 3, 7 and 11 o'clock positions
- Common causes:
    - chronic constipation
    - obstruction of rectal veins (due to pregnancy or portal HT)
- First-degree haemorrhoids:
    - in anal canal, produce PR bleeding
- Second-degree haemorrhoids:

  - prolapse on defaecation, but reduce spontaneously
- Third-degree haemorrhoids:
  - prolapse out of anal canal and require manual reduction
- Fourth-degree haemorrhoids:
  - irreducible
- Symptoms:
  - perianal itching (pruritus ani)
  - anal mass
  - PR bleeding
  - mucus discharge
  - pain (if thrombosis occurs)
- Investigations:
  - abdominal examination (masses and hepatomegaly)
  - PR examination
  - proctoscopy (first- and second-degree haemorrhoids can be seen)
  - sigmoidoscopy
- Complications:
  - strangulation (swell up and become blue-black in colour; cause severe pain)
- Management:
  - high-fibre diet
  - sclerotherapy using phenol in almond oil (for first- and second-degree haemorrhoids)
  - rubber banding ligation
  - closed haemorrhoidectomy (for third- and fourth-degree haemorrhoids)

Pruritus ani
- Causes:
  - threadworm infection
  - anorectal fistula/fissure
  - candidiasis
  - psoriasis
  - poor hygiene
- Symptoms:
  - itching
  - perineal pain
  - tenesmus
  - bleeding per rectum

Anal fissure
- Longitudinal tear in anal skin
- Mostly occurs in posterior midline
- Causes: injury while straining in constipation, Crohn's disease
- Symptoms: acute anal pain (tearing), mild anal bleeding
- Investigations:
  - proctoscopy

- – sigmoidoscopy
- Management:
  - – stool softeners
  - – in the case of small fissures, topical GTN cream to relax anal sphincter, allowing improvement in blood SS to fissure for healing to occur
  - – internal sphincterotomy

Fistula

= abnormal communication between two epithelial surfaces

- Common types of fistula:
  - – enterocutaneous
  - – colonic
  - – anorectal (fistula in ano)
  - – vesico-enteric
  - – vesico-vaginal
- Management:
  - – surgical excision

Hernia

- Common predisposing factors:
  - – constipation
  - – chronic cough
- Reducible, irreducible or strangulated
- Inguinal hernia: sac lies above and medial to pubic tubercle

Direct inguinal hernia (25%)

- Originates medial to inferior epigastric artery
- Does not pass through deep inguinal ring
- Due to weakness in transversalis fascia, pushes through fascia and is contained within aponeurosis of external oblique muscle

Indirect inguinal hernia (75%)

- Originates lateral to inferior epigastric artery
- Passes through deep inguinal ring
- Due to patent processus vaginalis, pushes through internal inguinal ring and may end up in scrotum
- Often repaired by surgery to eliminate the possibility of strangulation (which causes blood supply to structure to be cut off, resulting in ischaemia)

Femoral hernia (protrusion down femoral canal)

- Most commonly occurs in femoral ring (passes below inguinal lig.)
- Mostly seen in females
- Has high risk of strangulation and is irreducible (neck of femoral canal is narrow and has sharp border)
- Hernial sac lies below and lateral to pubic tubercle

5

Urinary system

- **Kidney**
  - vertebral level: T12–L3
  - developed from metanephric mesoderm (excretory parts) and ureteric bud (collecting duct)
  - surrounded by (from outermost to innermost layer) paranephric fat → renal fascia → perinephric fat → fibrous capsule
  - cortex, medulla, pyramids (tip of medullary pyramids = papillae), renal calyces, pelvis, ureter
  - nephron = basic structural and functional unit (contains glomerulus, proximal convoluted tubule (PCT), loop of Henlé, distal convoluted tubule (DCT) and collecting duct)
  - types of cells in glomerulus:
    - (i) endothelial cells
    - (ii) epithelial cells
    - (iii) mesangial cells – these cells have properties similar to smooth muscle cells and macrophages
  - glomerular basement membrane = basement membrane of endothelial cells + basement membrane of epithelial cells
- **Arterial SS (renal a.)**
  - segmental a.
  - lobar a.
  - interlobar a. (between pyramids)
  - arcuate a. (runs horizontally, to base of pyramids)
  - interlobular a. → afferent arterioles
- Venous drainage:
  - R. renal v. → IVC
  - L. renal v. → crosses ant. to aorta → IVC (longer course)
- Lymphatic drainage: para-aortic lymph nodes

- **Relationships of kidney**
  - medial: hilum (renal v., renal a. and pelvis of ureter)
  - ant.:
    R. kidney: second part of duodenum, ascending colon and liver
    L. kidney: descending colon, pancreas, spleen and stomach
  - post.: rib 12, transversus abdominis, diaphragm, psoas muscle
- Renal vessels have no collateral circulation → occlusion of any branch of renal a. → infarction
- R. renal a. passes post. to IVC
- **Proximal convoluted tubule (PCT)**
  - site of obligatory reabsorption and secretion
  - renal tubular cells (cuboidal epithelial cells with large amounts of mitochondria and brush border on surface for reabsorption of water and solutes)
- **Vasa recta**
  = capillaries that SS loop of Henlé
  - maintain concentration gradient
  - walls are freely permeable to water and solutes
- Juxtaglomerular apparatus:
  (a) macula densa cells of DCT
    - sense fall in GFR → release renin
  (b) granular cells of afferent arteriole
    - sense reduction in stretch of afferent arteriole → release renin
  (c) sympathetic renal nerves
    - release renin when blood pressure drops
- **Ureter (hilum of kidney → bladder)**
  - course: runs vertically down ant. to tips of transverse processes of lumbar vertebrae → runs down psoas major → crosses pelvic brim at bifurcation of common iliac a. ant. to sacro-iliac joint → runs downward and backward in pelvic cavity → spine of ischium → turns forward to run ant. to base of bladder → ureteric orifice
  - crossed by vas deferens in males
  - crossed by uterine a. in females
  - lined by transitional epithelium
  - sites of constrictions:
      (i) connection with renal pelvis
      (ii) cross pelvic brim
      (iii) connection with bladder wall
  - arterial SS:
      (i) U. part (renal a.)
      (ii) middle part (testicular/ovarian a.)
      (iii) L. part (sup. vesical a.)
- **Bladder**
  - sup. surface covered with peritoneum
  - pierced by ureters obliquely (prevents reflux of urine to kidneys)
  - trigone = smooth triangular area of mucosa between openings of ureters

on each side laterally
- in males, puboprostatic ligament connects neck of bladder to pelvis
- in females, pubovesical ligament connects neck of bladder to pelvis
- urachus runs from apex, and continues to umbilicus as medial umbilical ligament
- neck contains a large amount of elastic tissue (acts as internal sphincter)
- neck rests on prostate
- there are three layers of detrusor muscle
- arterial SS: vesicular branches from int. iliac a.
- parasym n. SS: S2–4; sym n. SS: T11–L2
- lymphatic drainage: int. and ext. iliac nodes
- **Relationships of bladder**
  - ant.: pubic symphysis
  - lat.: levator ani and obturator internus
  - post.: rectum in males, and vagina in females

Common pathologies

Horseshoe kidney
- Lower poles of kidney fuse in midline → single U-shaped kidney
- Ureters pass ant. to kidney
- Usually asymptomatic, but increased risk of kidney infections
- Can cause hydronephrosis

Polycystic kidney disease (PKD)
- Autosomal dominant polycystic kidney disease (ADPKD)
- Usually bilateral
- Risk factor: family history
- Symptoms:
  - abdominal discomfort
  - acute loin pain (haemorrhage into cysts)
  - haematuria
  - nocturia
  - HT
- Signs:
  - palpable kidneys
- Complications:
  - HT
  - formation of renal calculi
  - urinary tract infection
  - renal failure
- Investigations:
  - abdominal ultrasound scan
- Management:
  - hydration (to prevent development of kidney stones)

   – treat complications, including HT

Medullary sponge kidney
- Collecting ducts in medulla are dilated
- Cysts occur in papillae
- Symptoms:
  – pain if calculi form in cysts
  – haematuria
- Complications:
  – infections
  – formation of renal calculi

Alport's syndrome
- Congenital glomerular disease
- Associated with sensorineural deafness
- Symptoms:
  – haematuria
  – proteinuria
  – progressive renal failure
- Management:
  – ACE inhibitors

Glomerulonephritis
Diffuse (involves all glomeruli)
(a) Minimal change
- Mostly affects children
- Fusion of podocyte foot processes
- Responds to corticosteroid treatment

(b) Membranous nephropathy
- Thickening of glomerular basement membrane
- Circulating immune complexes
- Causes:
  – idiopathic
  – neoplasms (colon, lung)
  – infections (syphilis, malaria)
- Symptoms:
  – proteinuria
- Management:
  – administer alkylating agents (cyclophosphamide)

(c) Proliferative
- Mostly post-streptococcal infections
- Mostly affects children
- Symptoms: oliguria
- Increased blood urea levels
- Anti-streptolysin O (ASO) present in plasma

Focal (involves some glomeruli)
(a) IgA nephropathy
   • Symptoms:
      – haematuria
      – hypertension
   • Increased blood IgA levels
(b) Proliferative

Secondary (as part of systemic diseases)
(a) Goodpasture's syndrome
   • Antibodies against glomerular basement membrane
(b) Systemic lupus erythematosus (SLE)
(c) Infective endocarditis
(d) Diabetes mellitus
   • Leaky basement membrane
   • Symptoms: proteinuria
(e) Amyloidosis
   • Symptoms: proteinuria

Amyloidosis
– disorder of protein metabolism
• Protein deposits
• Amyloid stains red with Congo red dye

Acute tubular necrosis (ATN)
• Leads to acute renal failure
• Causes:
   (a) ischaemia
      – congestive heart failure
      – shock → hypotension → ischaemic injury to kidney
      – casts commonly found in collecting ducts
   (b) toxins
      – drugs (NSAIDs, aminoglycosides)
      – phenol
      – mainly affect proximal convoluted tubules
   (c) muscle injury
      – myoglobinaemia
      – haemoglobinaemia
• Symptoms:
   – oliguria
   – uraemia (pruritus, nausea, vomiting)

Nephritic syndrome
• General fluid retention
• Usually associated with hypertension
• Pathological feature: dysmorphic renal cells, red cell casts

- Causes: glomerulonephritis (post-streptococcal, post-infections, systemic lupus erythematosus, Henoch–Schönlein purpura)
- Symptoms:
  - oliguria
  - hypertension
  - haematuria
- Management:
  - treat HT
  - restrict sodium and fluid intake

Nephrotic syndrome
- Increased permeability of glomerular basement membrane to protein (albumin)
- Injury to podocytes
- Massive proteinuria and hypoalbuminaemia
- Usually associated with hyperlipidaemia
- Common causes:
  - glomerulonephritis
  - infections
  - systemic lupus erythematosus (SLE)
  - amyloidosis
  - diabetes mellitus
- Symptoms:
  - generalised oedema
- Investigations:
  - renal function tests
  - urine dipstick and culture
- Management:
  - diuretics
  - dietary changes (restriction of sodium and fluid intake)

Urinary tract calculi (kidney stones)
- Mostly composed of calcium oxalate
- Other types of stones:
  - calcium phosphate
  - ammonium phosphate
  - uric acid
  - mixed
- Risk factors:
  - urinary stasis (benign prostatic hypertrophy)
  - chronic urinary infection (*Proteus*)
  - low fluid intake
  - high sodium intake
  - hypercalcaemia
  - hyperoxaluria
  - cystinuria
  - medullary sponge kidney

- Symptoms:
  - renal colic (radiation from loin to groin)
  - loin pain
  - haematuria
- Complications:
  - pyelonephritis
  - urinary tract obstruction
  - hydronephrosis
  - renal failure
- Investigations:
  - AXR
  - blood tests
  - urine dipstick
  - MSU culture
  - IV pyelogram
  - ultrasound scan (may show dilation of ureter)
- Management:
  - percutaneous nephrostomy tube
  - shock-wave lithotripsy
  - endoscopic removal of stone

Urinary tract obstruction
- Causes:
  - (a) lumen wall
    - neuropathic bladder
    - stricture of ureter
  - (b) within lumen
    - tumour of ureter
    - tumour of renal pelvis
    - tumour of bladder
    - kidney calculus
  - (c) external pressure
    - pelvic tumour
    - diverticulitis
    - aortic aneurysm
- Symptoms:
  - loin pain (U. urinary tract)
  - sense of incomplete bladder emptying (L. urinary tract)
  - hesitancy (L. urinary tract)
- Investigations:
  - ultrasound scan
  - CT scan
- Management:
  - nephrostomy (drain urine)
  - surgery

Urinary tract infection (UTI)

- Most commonly involves bladder
- Most common organisms involved are *E. coli* from GI tract, *Saprophyticus* (in sexually active women) and *Proteus*
- Mostly spread from the urethra (which is short in women)
- U. tract: pyelonephritis
- L. tract: cystitis and urethritis
- Risk factors:
  - DM
  - prostatic hypertrophy
  - presence of kidney stones
  - dehydration
  - uterine prolapse
  - catheterisation
- Causes:
  - reflux of urine in bladder
  - spread from bloodstream
- Symptoms:
  - (a) U. urinary tract infection:
    - fever
    - nausea
    - vomiting
    - chills
    - unilat. pain in loin
  - (b) L. urinary tract infection:
    - fever
    - dysuria
    - frequency
    - haematuria
    - suprapubic pain
- Complications:
  - permanent kidney damage
  - pyonephrosis
  - may enter bloodstream (urosepsis)
- Investigations:
  - plasma urea and electrolytes
  - microscopy
  - MSU culture
  - urine dipstick
  - full blood count
- Management: antibiotic therapy (trimethoprim, ciprofloxacin)

Acute renal failure (ARF)

= rapid decline in renal function occurring over a period of hours or days (abrupt reduction in GFR)

- Causes:

(a) pre-renal:
  - hypovolaemia
  - HF
  - renal a. stenosis
  - renal a. thrombosis
(b) renal:
  - acute tubular necrosis
  - acute glomerulonephritis
  - malignant hypertension
  - nephrotoxic drugs (e.g. aminoglycosides) leading to acute interstitial nephritis
(c) post-renal:
  - kidney stones
  - prostatic hypertrophy
  - tumour obstructing both urine outflow tracts
- Characteristics:
  - fall in GFR
  - oliguria (urine output < 0.5 ml/kg/hour)
  - increase in serum creatinine concentration
- Investigations:
  - full blood count
  - blood urea, electrolytes, creatinine levels and BUN
  - MSU + urine microscopy and culture
  - urine dipstick
  - renal ultrasound scan (hydronephrosis)
- Management:
  (a) pre-renal:
    - replacement of fluid and electrolytes
    - loop diuretics
  (b) renal:
    - treat underlying cause
  (c) post-renal:
    - relieve obstruction
    - insert Foley catheter

Chronic renal failure (CRF)
- Scarring and loss of nephrons occurs
- Five stages (from mild to end-stage)
- Causes:
  - glomerulonephritis
  - hypertension
  - vasculitis
  - polycystic kidney disease
  - chronic pyelonephritis
  - amyloid deposits
  - diabetic glomerulosclerosis

- – thrombocytopenic purpura
- – TB
- – urinary tract obstruction
- Symptoms:
  - – nausea
  - – vomiting
  - – nocturia
  - – polyuria
  - – anaemia (due to reduction in release of erythropoietin)
  - – tetany (hypocalcaemia)
  - – pruritus
  - – confusion (severe uraemia)
  - – hypertension
  - – oedema
- Complications:
  - – anaemia
  - – acidosis
  - – sodium retention
  - – hyperkalaemia
  - – hyperuricaemia
  - – HT (due to increased production of renin)
  - – HF (due to cardiac overload), pulmonary oedema
  - – pruritus
  - – bone disease (renal osteodystrophy)
  - – gout (retention of urate)
- Investigations:
  - – blood tests (urea and creatinine)
  - – prothrombin time
  - – 24-hour urine
  - – urine microscopy and culture
  - – renal ultrasound scan
  - – renal biopsy
- Management:
  - – preserve function of existing nephrons (avoid nephrotoxic drugs, and correct fluid imbalances)
  - – restrict sodium and potassium intake
  - – control hypertension (diuretics)
  - – dialysis (haemodialysis, peritoneal dialysis)
  - – transplantation
  - – administer synthetic erythropoietin

Renal-cell carcinoma
- Risk factors:
  - – smoking
  - – HT
- Pathological findings: clear cells (tumour cells with clear cytoplasm)

- Symptoms:
  - haematuria
  - loin pain
  - renal mass
  - weight loss
  - malaise
- Paraneoplastic syndromes:
  - due to tumour secretion of renin, erythropoietin and parathyroid hormone-like substances
  - hypercalcaemia
  - HT (effect of renin)
  - amyloid deposition
  - polycythaemia
- Investigations:
  - full blood count
  - urinalysis
  - IV pyelogram
  - ultrasound scan
  - CT scan
- Management:
  - radical nephrectomy

Wilms' tumour
- Also known as nephroblastoma
- Usually seen in patients aged 1–3 years
- Pathological finding:
  - haemorrhagic necrosis
- Symptoms:
  - nausea
  - abnormal mass
  - haematuria
  - intestinal obstruction
  - hypertension
  - weight loss
- Signs:
  - painless abdominal mass
- Investigations:
  - excretion urography
- Management:
  - nephrectomy
  - chemotherapy
  - surgery

Exstrophy of bladder
- Bladder opens on to external surface of abdomen
- Can lead to pyelonephritis

Bladder cancer

- Mostly transitional-cell carcinoma (TCC)
- Can be adenocarcinoma or squamous-cell carcinoma
- Causes:
  - smoking
  - drugs
  - exposure to aniline dyes
- Symptoms:
  - painless haematuria
  - frequency
  - urgency
- Investigations:
  - midstream urine (MSU)
  - urinalysis
  - ultrasound scan of kidneys and bladder
  - KUB
  - IV pyelogram
  - cystoscopy with biopsy
- Management:
  - (a) superficial TCC: transurethral resection
  - (b) carcinoma *in situ*: immunotherapy
  - (c) invasive TCC: cystectomy/radiotherapy

6

Pelvis and perineum

- **Pelvis**
  - (a) Pelvic brim:
    - formed by sacral promontory (post.), iliopectineal lines and pubic symphysis
    - separates false pelvis (above) from true pelvis
  - (b) Pelvic outlet:
    - formed by coccyx, ischial tuberosities and pubic arch
    - contains sigmoid colon, rectum, ureters and bladder
- **Pelvic bone**
  - ilium (sup.) + ischium (post. + inf.) + pubis (ant.)
  - in anatomical position: anterior superior iliac spine + pubic tubercle lie in the same coronal plane
- **Ilium**
  - iliac crest: between ant. sup. iliac spine (ASIS) and post. sup. iliac spine (PSIS)
  - iliac tuberosity
  - ant. inf. iliac spine, post. inf. iliac spine
  - greater sciatic notch
  - lesser sciatic notch
  - ischial spine separates greater sciatic notch from lesser sciatic notch
  - sciatic notches are divided into greater and lesser sciatic foramina by sacrotuberous and sacrospinous ligaments
- **Ischium**
  - ischial spine (separates greater sciatic notch and lesser sciatic notch)
  - ischial tuberosity
  - ischial ramus
- **Pubis**
  - body
  - pubic tubercle

- pubic symphysis
- sup. pubic ramus
- inf. pubic ramus
- pubic crest
- **Differences between male and female pelvises**
  - female pelvis is wider between ischial spines and tuberosities
  - female pelvis inlet and outlet are wider
  - female pelvis inlet is oval-shaped
  - male pelvis inlet is heart-shaped
  - female pelvis has lighter bones
  - female pelvis has wider pubic arch (angle at pubic symphysis)
  - male pelvis has more prominent sacral promontory
- Iliopectineal line is continuous with pectineal line anteriorly and with arcuate line posteriorly.
- **Sacrotuberous ligament**
  - from lat. sacrum → ischial tuberosity
- **Sacrospinous ligament**
  - from lat. sacrum → ischial spine
- **Obturator foramen**
  - bounded by ischium and pubis
  - partly covered by obturator membrane
  - uncovered part = obturator canal
- **Levator ani muscle**
  - function: supports pelvic viscera
  (a) Puborectalis:
  - origin: pubis
  - insertion: sling around anal aperture
  - nerve SS: inf. rectal branch of pudendal n. (S2–4)
  (b) Pubococcygeus:
  - origin: body of pubis
  - insertion: coccyx
  - nerve SS: inf. rectal branch of pudendal n. (S2–4)
  (c) Iliococcygeus:
  - origin: fascia overlying obturator internus
  - insertion: joins iliococcygeus on other side
  - nerve SS: inf. rectal branch of pudendal n. (S2–4)
- **Attachments of iliacus**
  - origin: iliac fossa
  - insertion: lesser trochanter of femur
  - nerve SS: femoral n. (L2–4)
  - function: flex and laterally rotate thigh
- **Attachments of piriformis muscle**
  - origin: ant. sacrum
  - insertion: greater trochanter of femur
  - nerve SS: n. to piriformis (S1 and 2)
  - function: laterally rotate hip

- **Attachments of obturator internus muscle**
  - origin: obturator membrane and ischiopubic ramus
  - insertion: medial part of greater trochanter of femur
  - nerve SS: n. to obturator internus (L5–S2)
  - function: laterally rotate hip
- **Branches of ext. iliac a.**
  - deep circumflex iliac a.
  - inf. epigastric a.
- **Branches of int. iliac a.**
  - (a) ant. trunk:
    - obturator a.
    - umbilical a.
    - inf. vesical a.
    - middle rectal a.
    - int. pudendal a.
    - uterine a.
    - inf. gluteal a.
    - vaginal a.
  - (b) post. trunk:
    - sup. gluteal a.
    - ilio-lumbar a.
    - lat. sacral a.
- **Perineum**
  - diamond-shaped when seen inferiorly; line drawn between ischial tuberosities divides perineum into ant. and post. parts
  - ant. part = urogenital triangle
  - post. part = anal triangle
- **Anal canal**
  - ant. to anococcygeal body
  - bounded by ischiorectal fossae laterally
  - outer longitudinal smooth muscle and inner circular smooth muscle
  - divided into U. + L. halves by pectinate line
  - U. half lined by columnar epithelium (SS by sup. rectal a.) (no SS by somatic n. → no pain sensation)
  - contains anal columns
  - L. half lined by stratified squamous epithelium (SS by inf. rectal a.)
  - dentate line = midpoint of anal canal
  - lymphatic drainage:
    - (i) U. half drains to pelvic and abdominal lymph nodes
    - (ii) L. half drains to inguinal lymph nodes
- **Anal sphincter**
  - (a) External sphincter:
    - skeletal muscle
    - blends with puborectalis to form anorectal ring
  - (b) Internal sphincter:
    - smooth muscle

- involuntary
- **Ischiorectal fossae**
  - lie on each side of anal canal
  - medial wall = levator ani
  - lateral wall = obturator internus
  - posterior wall = sacrotuberous ligament
  - contents:
    - (i) fat
    - (ii) pudendal n.
    - (iii) internal pudendal a.
    - (iv) internal pudendal v.
    - (v) inf. rectal a.
    - (vi) inf. rectal v.
    - (vii) inf. rectal n.
  - infection can spread from one fossa to the other
- **Urogenital triangle**
  - boundaries:
    - (i) pubic arch ant.
    - (ii) ischiopubic rami lat.
    - (iii) line between ischial tuberosities post.
  - contents:
    - (i) penis and scrotum in males
    - (ii) external genitalia, urethral opening and vagina in females
  - urogenital diaphragm = superior fascial layer + sphincter urethrae + inferior fascial layer (perineal membrane)
  - perineal membrane is pierced by urethra in males and by urethra and vagina in females
- **Superficial perineal pouch**
  - superior boundary = urogenital diaphragm
  - inferior boundary = membranous layer of superficial fascia (Colles' fascia)
  - lateral boundary = pubic arch
- **Structures in superficial perineal pouch in males**
  - root of penis
  - bulbospongiosus
  - ischiocavernosus
  - superficial transverse perineal muscle
- **Structures in superficial perineal pouch in females**
  - root of clitoris
  - bulbospongiosus
  - ischiocavernosus
  - superficial transverse perineal muscle
- **Attachments of ischiocavernosus**
  - origin: ischial tuberosity and ramus
  - insertion: crus of penis in males or clitoris in females
  - nerve SS: pudendal n. (S2–4)
- **Attachments of bulbospongiosus**

- – origin: perineal body
- – insertion: corpus cavernosum
- – nerve SS: pudendal n. (S2–4)
- **Attachments of superficial transverse perineal muscle**
  - – origin: ischial tuberosity and ramus
  - – insertion: perineal body
  - – nerve SS: pudendal n. (S2–4)
- **Deep perineal pouch**
  - – superior to inferior fascial layer of urogenital diaphragm
- **Structures in deep perineal pouch in males**
  - – dorsal n. of penis
  - – internal pudendal a. (a. to bulb of penis, a. to crura of penis, dorsal a. of penis)
  - – external urethral sphincter
  - – bulbourethral glands
  - – membranous urethra
  - – deep transverse perineal muscle
- **Structures in deep perineal pouch in females**
  - – external urethral sphincter
  - – compressor urethrae
  - – deep transverse perineal muscle
- **Coccygeal plexus**
  - – descending branch of S4, ventral primary rami of S5, coccygeal spinal n.
  - – gives off cutaneous branches that innervate perineal skin ant. to coccyx

7

Male reproductive system

- **Scrotum**
  - fat in superficial fascia is replaced by dartos muscle (SS by sympathetic n.)
  - membranous layer in superficial fascia (Colles' fascia) is continuous with Scarpa's fascia of abdominal wall
  - arterial SS: ext. pudendal branches of femoral a. and scrotal branches of int. pudendal a.
  - lymphatic drainage: para-aortic nodes
- **Testes**
  - produce sperm and sex hormones
  - lie within scrotum
  - surrounded by capsule (tunica albuginea)
  - descent occurs in last 2 months of fetal development (if not: cryptorchidism)
  - divided into lobules (contains seminiferous tubules = site where spermatogenesis occurs)
  - seminiferous tubules → rete testes → efferent ductules → head of epididymis → tail of epididymis
  - interstitial cells lie between seminiferous tubules (secrete androgens such as testosterone)
  - arterial SS: testicular a. (from abdominal aorta)
  - venous drainage: L. testicular v. (drains to L. renal vein)
                                R. testicular v. (drains to IVC)
  - lymphatic drainage: para-aortic lymph nodes
  - nerve SS: T10 sympathetic fibres
- **Epididymis**
  - coiled tube that lies post. to testes
  - parts: head, body and tail → emerges as vas deferens

- groove between testes and epididymis is lined with tunica vaginalis = sinus of epididymis
- stores spermatozoa, allows maturation to take place, absorbs fluid, and contributes to formation of seminal fluid
- arterial SS: testicular a.
- venous drainage: pampiniform plexus
- **Vas deferens**
  - transports sperm from tail of epididymis
  - forms part of spermatic cord
  - joins seminal vesicle to form ejaculatory duct
  - opens into prostatic urethra
- **Course of vas deferens (direct continuation of epididymis)**
  - runs in spermatic cord (passes through inguinal canal) → deep inguinal ring → crosses pelvic brim → downward and backward to base of bladder → crosses lat. wall of pelvic cavity → crosses above and medial to ureter → becomes ampulla of vas deferens
- **Seminal vesicle**
  - extraperitoneal structure
  - anatomical relationships:
    - (i) post. to bladder
    - (ii) lat. to end of vas deferens
    - (iii) ant. to rectum
    - (iv) duct of seminal vesicle joins with vas deferens to form ejaculatory duct → enters post. part of prostate
  - contributes to formation of seminal fluid (provides nutrients for spermatozoa)
- **Male urethra**
  - (a) prostatic urethra (widest part)
    - urethral crest on post. wall
  - (b) membranous urethra (surrounded by ext. urethral sphincter)
  - (c) spongy urethra
    - runs along corpus spongiosum of penis
- **Prostate**
  - encapsulated by fibrous capsule
  - ant. + post. + middle + two lat. lobes
  - contains post. median sulcus
  - central zone (25%) + peripheral zone (75%) (usual site of carcinoma)
  - connected to ejaculatory ducts (opens through prostatic utricle) posteriorly
  - sandwiched between neck of bladder and urogenital diaphragm
  - contributes to formation of seminal fluid (alkaline secretion)
  - arterial SS: inf. vesical a. (from int. iliac a.)
  - venous drainage: prostatic venous plexus

- **Relationships of prostate**
  - ant.: pubic symphysis
  - lat.: levator ani
  - post.: rectum
  - sup.: neck of bladder
- **Bulbourethral glands (Cowper's glands)**
  - mucous glands in deep perineal pouch
  - on either side of urethra
  - contribute to formation of seminal fluid
- **Penis (root and body)**
  - root: bulb of penis + R. crus + L. crus
  - bulb continues as corpus spongiosum
  - crura continue as corpora cavernosa
  - body: two corpora cavernosa (dorsal aspect) + corpus spongiosum (ventral aspect)
  - corpus spongiosum expands distally → glans penis (covered by foreskin)
  - arterial SS:
    - (i) dorsal a. of penis
    - (ii) deep a. of penis (SS corpora cavernosa)
    - (iii) a. of bulb (SS corpora spongiosum) (all from internal pudendal a.)
  - venous drainage: internal pudendal veins

Common pathologies

Klinefelter's syndrome
- 47XXY
- Hypogonadism
- Clinical features:
  - small testes
  - type 2 diabetes
- Investigations:
  - karyotype analysis

Prostatitis
= inflammatory disorder of prostate

Acute prostatitis
- Symptoms:
  - fever
  - perineal pain
  - frequency
- Investigations:
  - rectal examination
- Management:
  - antibiotics

Chronic prostatitis
- Symptoms:
  - dull suprapubic pain
- Management:
  - antibiotics
  - anti-inflammatory drugs

Benign prostatic hyperplasia (BPH)
- Affects lat. lobes of prostate
- Nodular hyperplasia of glands and stroma
- Peri-urethral zone involved
- Urethra compressed
- Symptoms:
  - urinary retention (pain)
  - hesitancy
  - frequency
  - urgency
- Complications:
  - bladder diverticula
  - pyelonephritis
  - bilateral hydronephrosis
  - renal failure
- Investigations:
  - urea and electrolytes
  - rectal examination
  - ultrasound scan
  - CT scan
  - cystoscopy
- Management:
  - urethral catheterisation
  - 5-alpha-reductase inhibitors (finasteride)
  - transurethral resection of prostate (TURP)

Prostate cancer
- Adenocarcinoma
- Most commonly occurs in men aged 65–85 years
- Aetiology uncertain
- Mostly androgen dependent
- Sites of origin (in decreasing order of frequency):
  - from peripheral zone
  - from transition zone
  - from central zone
- Median groove obliterated in posterior subcapsular zone
- Usually metastasises to bone
- Can spread through stromal invasion, via lymphatics or via bloodstream
- Symptoms:

- bladder outlet obstruction (hesitancy, acute retention, poor stream, nocturia)
- haematuria
- back pain
- weight loss
- lethargy
- metastatic (bone pain, jaundice)
- Investigations:
  - blood tests for serum tumour marker PSA (prostate-specific antigen) (a concentration of > 10 ng/ml suggests prostate cancer, but PSA levels can also increase in BPH)
  - cystoscopy
  - digital rectal examination (DRE)
  - pelvic CT/MRI (staging)
  - bone scan (metastases)
  - ultrasound scan
  - CXR (lung metastases)
- Management:
  - radical prostatectomy
  - radiotherapy
  - hormonal therapy (anti-androgen: cyproterone acetate, luteinising-hormone-releasing hormone (LHRH) agonists)

Cryptorchidism
= undescended testes
- Testes remain outside scrotum
- Can increase risk of tumour development
- Management: surgery

Spermatocoele
- Swelling in epididymis
- Caused by obstruction in vas deferens
- Spermatic cord is palpable above swelling

Varicocoele
- More common on LHS
- Varicosity of pampiniform plexus of veins around spermatic cord
- May be due to malfunction of valves in veins
- Causes infertility
- Symptoms:
  - scrotal swelling
  - veins tortuous and dilated
- Management:
  - ligation of testicular vein

Torsion of spermatic cord
- Urological emergency
- Usually occurs within tunica vaginalis
- Symptoms: severe pain
- Investigations: Doppler ultrasound scan
- Complications: testicular a. may be occluded → testicular necrosis

Hypospadias
- Congenital condition
- Caused by failure of fusion of urethral fold over urogenital sinus
- Urethral opening on ventral aspect of penis
- Commonly occurs on inferior aspect of glans
- Can occur on shaft of penis

Epispadias
- Less common than hypospadias
- Urethral opening on dorsal aspect of penis
- Commonly occurs at base of shaft of penis
- Associated with exstrophy of bladder

Orchitis
= inflammation of testes

Syphilitic orchitis
= painless enlargement of testes

Mumps orchitis
= painful enlargement of testes

Hydrocoele
= accumulation of fluid in tunica vaginalis of testes
- Can be transilluminated
- Symptoms: painless scrotal swelling

Congenital hydrocoele
- Due to persistent tunica vaginalis

Secondary hydrocoele
- Due to lesion of testes/epididymis
- Investigations:
  - ultrasound scan
- Management:
  - surgery
  - aspiration of fluid
- Complications:
  - compression of testicular blood SS

Haematocoele

= haemorrhage into tunica vaginalis
- Cannot be transilluminated
- Testes will be compressed
- Causes:
  - testicular tumour
  - trauma
- Symptoms:
  - painfull scrotal swelling
- Management:
  - analgesics
  - surgery

Testicular tumour

Germ-cell tumours

(a) Seminoma
  - Most common
  - Arise from seminiferous tubules
  - Radiosensitive
(b) Teratoma
  - Aggressive
  - Arise from germ cells

Non-germ-cell tumours

(a) Leydig cell tumours
(b) Lymphoma
  - Symptoms:
    - firm painless lump in testicular region
    - gynaecomastia
  - Signs:
    - retroperitoneal mass
  - Investigations:
    - blood tests (AFP, HCG)
    - ultrasound scan
    - CT scan for staging
  - Management:
    - surgical orchidectomy
    - radiotherapy
    - chemotherapy (for metastatic diseases)
  - Metastasise through lymphatics to para-aortic nodes
  - Lung metastases are common

8

Female reproductive system

- **Broad ligament**
  - runs between lat. uterus → pelvic walls
  - mesosalpinx = part of broad ligament between mesovarium and uterine tube
  - superior margin contains uterine tube
  - contents:
    - (i) ovary
    - (ii) ovarian ligament
    - (iii) Fallopian tube
    - (iv) round ligament
    - (v) uterine and ovarian vessels
    - (vi) nerves and lymphatics
- **Ovaries**
  - produces ova (oogenesis) and sex hormones (oestrogen and progesterone)
  - attached to pelvic wall by broad ligament (posteriorly)
  - attached to broad ligament by mesovarium
  - attached to uterus by ovarian ligament
  - arterial SS: ovarian a. (branch from abdominal aorta)
  - venous drainage:
    RHS: IVC
    LHS: L. renal vein
  - lymphatic drainage: para-aortic nodes
- **Fallopian tube**
  - infundibulum + ampulla (widest part; usual site of fertilisation) + isthmus (narrowest part) + intramural part
  - transports ova to uterus
  - infundibulum contains fimbriae that sweep over ovary during ovulation to transport egg into tube

  – lined by cilia that propel egg to uterus
- **Uterus**
  – myometrium lined by endometrium (forms placenta)
  – fundus (lies above openings to Fallopian tubes) + body + cervix
  – arterial SS: uterine a. (branch of int. iliac a.) (crosses above ureter)
  – venous drainage: uterine vein
  – lymphatic drainage: para-aortic nodes and ext. iliac nodes
- **Cervix**
  – inf. part of uterus
  – angled forward on vagina
  – continuous with uterus body through internal os
  – continuous with vagina through external os
- **Vagina**
  – birth canal + receives penis during copulation
  – ant. + post. + lat. fornices
  – arterial SS: vaginal a. (int. iliac a.) + vaginal branch of uterine a.
  – venous drainage: vaginal veins (int. iliac v.)
  – lymphatic drainage:
     (i) U. third to ext. and int. iliac nodes
     (ii) middle third to int. iliac nodes
     (iii) L. third to superficial inguinal nodes
- Relationships of vagina
  – ant.: bladder
  – lat.: levator ani
  – post.: rectum, anal canal
- **External genitalia (vulva)**
  – mons pubis: fatty pad overlying pubic symphysis
  – labia majora
  – labia minora: form prepuce ant.
  – clitoris
  – vestibule: cleft between labia minora; contains urethral + vaginal + greater vestibular gland openings

Common pathologies

Pelvic inflammatory disease (PID)
= inflammation of Fallopian tubes, endometrium and pelvic peritoneum
- Risk factors:
  – use of intrauterine devices (IUDs)
  – history of salpingitis
- Symptoms:
  – vaginal discharge
  – pelvic pain
- Signs:
  – fever

– abdominal tenderness
- Investigations:
  – blood tests (raised WCC)
  – cervical culture
  – laparoscopy
- Complications:
  – tubo-ovarian abscess
  – infertility
- Management:
  – antibiotics
  – surgery (if complications occur)

Turner's syndrome
- 45XO karyotype
- Fibrosis of ovaries → 'streak ovaries'
- Clinical features:
  – abnormal LFTs
  – type 2 diabetes
  – short stature
  – hypertension
  – webbed neck
  – swollen hands and feet
  – psychological problems
  – coarctation of aorta
  – reduced bone density
- Investigations:
  – karyotype analysis
- Management:
  – growth hormone for short stature

Ovarian cysts
- Can be non-neoplastic or neoplastic

Polycystic ovary syndrome
- Associated with hyperoestrogenism and amenorrhoea
- Clinical features:
  – excess androgen (causes acne and hirsutism)
  – loss of control of menstrual cycle (causes oligomenorrhoea and amenorrhoea)
- Causes infertility
- Management:
  – anti-androgen drugs (cyproterone acetate, spironolactone)

Ovarian cancer
- Can originate from any of the following:
  (a) epithelial cells (most common primary):

  - serous type
  - mucinous type
  - endometrioid type
  - clear cell type
  (b) germ cells:
  - dysgerminoma
  - teratoma
  (c) sex-cord stroma:
  - thecoma
  - granulosa-cell tumour
  (d) metastatic tumours
- Risk factors:
  - breast cancer
  - family history
- Symptoms:
  - GU symptoms
  - mostly asymptomatic until later stages
  - lower abdominal pain
- Investigations:
  - α-fetoprotein (germ-cell cancers)
  - abdominal CT
- Management:
  - surgery followed by chemotherapy

Salpingitis
= inflammation of Fallopian tube
- Causes:
  - placement of intrauterine device
  - infection of endometrium by anaerobic organisms

Bicornuate uterus
- Congenital abnormality
- Two uterine cavities and one vaginal opening

Endometrial cancer
- Mostly adenocarcinoma
- Risk factors:
  - early menarche
  - endometrial hyperplasia
  - diabetes mellitus
- Symptoms:
  - palpable abdominal mass
  - postmenopausal uterine bleeding
- Investigations:
  - endometrial biopsy
- Management:

- hysterectomy
- radiotherapy
- chemotherapy

Endometrial adenocarcinoma

There are two types:

(a) endometrioid adenocarcinoma
- due to unopposed oestrogen stimulation
- usually occurs in young women with polycystic ovaries

(b) non-endometrioid adenocarcinoma
- not associated with oestrogen stimulation
- usually occurs in elderly postmenopausal women
- spreads through lymphatic ducts and bloodstream

Endometriosis

= proliferation of endometrial tissue in organs other than the endometrial cavity

- Risk factors:
  - age > 25 years
  - family history
- Common sites:
  - ovaries
  - wall of vagina
  - rectosigmoid colon
  - bladder
- Recurrent haemorrhage in ovary may produce cysts with altered blood contents, known as 'chocolate cysts'
- Symptoms:
  - pelvic pain
  - menorrhagia
  - dysmenorrhoea
  - GI symptoms (diarrhoea, haematochezia)
  - bladder symptoms (dysuria, haematuria)
- Complications:
  - pelvic inflammation
  - infertility
- Investigations:
  - laparoscopy
  - ultrasound scan
- Management:
  - medical treatment
  - surgery (in serious cases)

Endometrial cancer

- Most commonly adenocarcinoma
- Risk factors:

- early menarche
- endometrial hyperplasia
- diabetes mellitus
- Symptoms:
  - palpable abdominal mass
  - postmenopausal uterine bleeding
- Investigations:
  - endometrial biopsy
- Management:
  - hysterectomy
  - radiotherapy
  - chemotherapy

Hydatidiform mole
- Placental abnormality
- Swollen chorionic villi
- Trophoblastic hyperplasia
- Associated with high hCG levels
- Clinical features:
  - anaemia
  - bleeding during early pregnancy
- Complications:
  - uterine perforation
  - choriocarcinoma
(a) Partial mole
  - can be XXX, XXY or XYY
  - fetus may be present
(b) Complete mole
  - most common type
  - 46XX
  - fetus is not present

Ectopic pregnancy
= implantation of fertilised ovum outside endometrial cavity
- Most common site is Fallopian tube
- Risk factors:
  - previous ectopic pregnancy
  - use of intrauterine device
- Rupture commonly occurs → haematoperitoneum and pain
- Classical presentation:
  - female of reproductive age presenting with acute hypotension, acute abdomen, vaginal bleeding and amenorrhoea
- Signs:
  - guarding
  - severe tenderness
- Referred pain to shoulder may occur if there is irritation of the

subdiaphragmatic peritoneum
- Investigations:
  - ultrasound scan
  - laparoscopy

Cervical cancer

- Most commonly caused by human papillomavirus (HPV)
- Risk factors:
  - multiple sexual partners
  - smoking
  - family history
- Usually occurs in transformation zone (squamo-columnar junction)
- Usually squamous-cell carcinoma
- Symptoms:
  - postcoital bleeding
- Investigations:
  - Pap smear
- Management:
  - surgery, chemotherapy or radiotherapy, depending on stage

9

Endocrine system

- **Ant. pituitary gland (adenohypophysis)**
  - fenestrated capillary walls
  - upgrowth from roof of mouth (Rathke's pouch)
  - pars tuberalis + pars intermedia + pars anterior
  - primary and secondary plexus + intervening hypophyseal portal vein = hypophyseal portal system
  - hormones produced: GH, TSH, ACTH, FSH, LH and prolactin
- **Post. pituitary gland (neurohypophysis)**
  - median eminence + neural stalk + pars nervosa
  - downgrowth of hypothalamic tissue (maintains neural connection with hypothalamus via neural bundle)
  - hypothalamic–hypophyseal tract (arises from supraoptic and paraventricular nuclei of hypothalamus)
- **Structure of thyroid**
  - R. and L. lobe
  - pyramidal lobe (present in 50% of patients)
  - isthmus (ant. to tracheal rings 2–4)
  - covered by pre-tracheal fascia (attaches gland to trachea and larynx post.)
- **Blood supply to thyroid**
  - superior thyroid artery (from external carotid a.)
  - inferior thyroid artery (from thyrocervical trunk of subclavian a.)
  - thyroidea ima artery (may be present) (from aortic arch)
- **Venous drainage of thyroid**
  - superior and middle thyroid v. → IJV
  - inferior thyroid v. → brachiocephalic veins
- **Nerves at risk during thyroid surgery**
  - superior laryngeal nerve (SLN)
  - recurrent laryngeal nerve (RLN)

- RLN passes under subclavian a. → goes back up in groove between oesophagus and trachea
  - LLN passes under arch of aorta → goes back up in groove between oesophagus and trachea
  - RLN and LLN in close association with inf. thyroid a.
  - RLN innervates laryngeal intrinsic muscles and gives sensory supply to mucous membrane below vocal folds → hoarseness if unilateral damage occurs and airway obstruction if bilateral damage occurs
- External laryngeal nerve runs alongside superior thyroid a. Recurrent laryngeal nerves closely associated with inferior thyroid a.
- **Parathyroid (post. to thyroid)**
  - inferior parathyroid originates from third branchial pouch with thymus (thymus descends, dragging inf. parathyroid with it)
  - superior parathyroid originates from fourth branchial pouch
  - arterial SS: inf. thyroid a.
  - chief cells produce PTH (increases blood calcium levels, decreases blood phosphate levels)
  - oxyphil cells (function unclear)
- **Thymus**
  - deep to sternum
  - mostly adipose and fibrous connective tissue in adult
  - produces thymopoietins and thymosins (development of T-lymphocytes, which promote growth of peripheral lymphoid tissue)
- **Adrenal gland**
  - lies on U. pole of kidneys
  - cortex (derived from mesoderm) and medulla (derived from ectoderm)
  - cortex has three layers:
    - (i) zona glomerulosa (aldosterone)
    - (ii) zona fasciculata (androgens and cortisol)
    - (iii) zona reticularis (oestrogen, androgens and cortisol)
- **Arterial SS of adrenal gland**
  - inferior phrenic artery
  - renal artery
  - aorta
- **Venous drainage of adrenal gland**
  - Right: IVC
  - Left: renal vein

Common pathologies

Pituitary tumours
- Mostly prolactinoma or non-secreting pituitary tumour
- Can also be tumours of somatotroph, corticotroph, gonadotroph or thyrotroph
- Investigations:
  - skull X-ray

- CT scan (enlarged pituitary fossa)
- MRI
- pituitary stimulation tests

Prolactinoma
- Manifestation in males:
  - impotence
  - reduced libido
- Manifestation in females:
  - galactorrhoea
  - infertility
  - amenorrhoea

Growth hormone deficiency
- Symptoms in children:
  - reduced growth rate
  - reduced height
- Symptoms in adults:
  - obesity
  - reduced muscle strength
  - raised levels of cholesterol

Growth hormone hypersecretion
- Causes acromegaly (enlargement of facial features and hands and feet)
- Eosinophil adenoma

Gonadotrophin deficiency
- Symptoms in males:
  - impotence
  - testicular atrophy
  - reduced libido
- Symptoms in females:
  - reduced libido
  - amenorrhoea
- Symptoms in children:
  - delayed puberty

Cushing's disease
- Cushing's syndrome is caused by excessive production of ACTH by ant. pituitary gland
- Basophil adenoma
- Symptoms:
  - striae
  - truncal obesity
  - easy bruising
  - proximal myopathy
  - weight gain
- Investigations:

- high-dose dexamethasone suppression test
- Management:
  - trans-sphenoidal adenomectomy

Panhypopituitarism
- Usually caused by pituitary adenoma
- Deficiency of several ant. pituitary hormones

Thyrotrophin deficiency
- Symptoms:
  - constipation
  - fatigue
  - cold intolerance
  - weight gain

Acromegaly
- Clinical features:
  - hypertension
  - headache
  - increased risk of cardiomyopathy and colon cancer
  - enlarged lips and tongue
  - enlarged liver
  - carpal tunnel syndrome
  - protruding lower jaw
  - thick skin
  - enlarged hands and feet
  - myopathy
- Investigations: GH levels in oral glucose tolerance test
- Management:
  - surgery
  - radiotherapy

Hyperprolactinaemia
- Causes:
  - drug induced (anti-emetics, antipsychotics)
  - pregnancy
  - lactation
  - oral contraceptive pill
  - prolactinoma
  - hypothyroidism
  - polycystic ovary syndrome
  - pituitary tumour
- Investigations:
  - MRI of the pituitary gland
- Management:
  - dopamine agonist (bromocriptine)
  - surgery through trans-sphenoidal approach

Hashimoto's thyroiditis
- Autoimmune disease
- Thyroid infiltrated with lymphocytes
- Antithyroid Ab found in serum
- Gradual atrophy and fibrosis of thyroid
- Symptoms:
  - mostly euthyroid
  - hypothyroid at later stages
  - diffuse thyroid enlargement
  - tender thyroid
- Investigations:
  - antithyroid Ab
- Management:
  - oral thyroxine

Palpable nodules
- Cold or hot (increased or decreased ^{121}I uptake)
- Cold nodules have higher risk of malignancy
- Ultrasound scan differentiates between solid and cystic nodules
- Investigations: ultrasound-guided fine-needle aspiration (FNA)

Hypothyroidism
- If congenital, causes cretinism (impaired growth and mental development)
- Causes:
  - congenital
  - low levels of iodine in diet
  - surgical removal of thyroid gland
  - overdose of antithyroid drugs
  - autoimmune disease (Hashimoto's disease)
  - anterior pituitary disorder (TSH deficiency) (secondary hypothyroidism)
- Symptoms:
  - cold intolerance
  - weight gain
  - dry, cold skin
  - hoarse voice
  - lethargy
  - delayed ankle reflex
  - carpal tunnel syndrome
  - reduced libido
  - myalgia
  - oligomenorrhoea
  - constipation
- Signs:
  - psychosis
  - loss of lat. third of eyebrow
  - bradycardia

- oedema
- obesity
- slow reflexes
- Investigations:
  - blood tests (hyponatraemia, anaemia)
  - thyroid function tests (reduced free and total T4, increased TSH)
  - ultrasound scan
- Management:
  - replacement hormones (thyroxine)

Thyrotoxicosis
- Excess thyroid hormones in circulation
- Mostly due to Graves' disease or toxic nodular goitre
- Other causes:
  - thyroiditis
  - drug induced
- Symptoms:
  - heat intolerance
  - vomiting
  - tachycardia
  - restlessness
  - tremor
  - weight loss despite normal appetite
  - fatigue
  - oligomenorrhoea
- Signs:
  - psychosis
  - warm peripheries
  - lid lag
  - exophthalmos
  - goitre
  - onycholysis
  - pretibial myxoedema
- Investigations:
  - thyroid function tests
- Management:
  - antithyroid drugs (carbimazole, propylthiouracil)
  - radioactive iodide therapy
  - thyroidectomy
- Complications:
  - thyroid storm

Graves' disease
- Autoimmune disorder
- Circulating long-acting thyroid immunoglobulin (LATI) that mimics TSH
- Ab produced stimulates thyroid

- Symptoms: diffusely enlarged gland
- Signs:
  - heat intolerance
  - thyroid acropachy
  - muscle weakness
  - exophthalmos
  - lid lag
  - tremor
  - goitre
  - tachycardia
  - palpitations
  - weight loss
  - fatigue
- Pathology: hyperplastic follicles
- Investigations: thyroid function tests
- Management:
  - total thyroidectomy
  - antithyroid drugs

Thyroid storm

- Life-threatening condition
- Symptoms:
  - tachycardia
  - confusion
  - fever
  - atrial fibrillation
- Management:
  - broad-spectrum antibiotic
  - propranolol

Thyroid cancer

- Major types of thyroid cancer (in decreasing order of frequency)
  - (a) papillary adenocarcinoma (80%)
    - 'Orphan Annie' nuclei
    - good prognosis
  - (b) follicular adenocarcinoma (aggressive)
    - single encapsulated lesion
    - usually spread to bone
  - (c) medullary adenocarcinoma (aggressive)
    - derived from thyroid parafollicular C-cells
    - usually have cervical lymphadenopathy
    - associated with multiple endocrine neoplasia type 2
  - (d) anaplastic carcinoma
  - (e) thyroid lymphoma
- Risk factors:
  - neck radiation

- family history of thyroid cancer
- Symptoms:
  - dysphagia
  - neck discomfort due to compression on trachea and oesophagus
  - hoarseness of voice
- Signs:
  - lymphadenopathy
  - neck mass
  - mostly euthyroid
- Investigations:
  - fine-needle aspiration (FNA)
  - radionuclide thyroid scan
  - ultrasound scan of thyroid gland
  - serum TSH level

Toxic multinodular goitre

= multiple thyroid nodules, some producing thyroid hormone →
hyperthyroidism
- Investigations:
  - thyroid function tests
  - fine-needle aspiration
  - ultrasound scan with high resolution
- Management:
  - surgical resection of hyperfunctioning nodules
  - thyroidectomy
  - radioiodine

Hypoparathyroidism (fall in serum calcium levels)
- Most common cause: surgical removal of parathyroid glands during total thyroidectomy
- Other causes: congenital deficiency
- Symptoms:
  - tetany
  - convulsions
- Chvostek's sign (tapping over site of facial nerve induces contraction of facial muscles)
- Investigations:
  - blood tests (plasma PTH low or absent)
- Management:
  - IV calcium for acute cases

Primary hyperparathyroidism

= secretion of inappropriately large amount of parathyroid hormone (PTH) by
parathyroid glands
- Causes:
  - single adenoma of parathyroid (most cases)

- hyperplasia of parathyroid
- parathyroid cancer
- Risk factors:
  - family history
  - MEN-I
  - MEN-II
- Usually high calcium and PTH levels and low phosphorus levels in blood
- Clinical presentation:
  - kidney stones
  - bone resorption leading to bone pain
  - muscle pain and weakness
  - polyuria
  - peptic ulcer
  - depression

Secondary hyperparathyroidism
= compensatory excessive secretion of PTH due to hypocalcaemia
- Causes:
  - chronic renal failure: poor kidney excretion of phosphate causes a reduction in serum calcium levels (most common cause)
  - malabsorption
  - renal tubular acidosis
  - osteomalacia
- Pathology: chief cell hyperplasia
- Usually low calcium levels in blood with raised PTH

Tertiary hyperparathyroidism
= development of hypersecreting adenoma with background secondary hyperparathyroidism

Parathyroid cancer
- Signs:
  - hypercalcaemia
  - elevated PTH
  - palpable parathyroid gland
- Tumour marker: human chorionic gonadotrophin (HCG)
- Management: surgical resection of parathyroid

Hypercalcaemia
- Causes:
  - with raised PTH: primary hyperparathyroidism
  - with low PTH: malignant hypercalcaemia (tumours in ovary, lung, colon and breast)
- Symptoms:
  - lethargy

- peptic ulcer
- impaired cognition
- polydipsia
- polyuria
- nausea
- constipation

Diabetes mellitus (DM)
- Macrovascular complications:
  - intermittent claudication
  - transient ischaemic attack (TIA)
  - stroke
  - MI
- Microvascular complications:
  - peripheral neuropathy
  - autonomic neuropathy
  - foot ulceration
  - renal failure
  - retinopathy

Type 1 DM (insulin-dependent)
- Also called juvenile-onset diabetes
- Cause: development of antibodies against pancreatic islet cells → loss of pancreatic beta cells
- Autoimmune disease
- Symptoms:
  - polyuria
  - polydipsia
  - weight loss
  - blurred vision
  - nocturia
- Investigations:
  - plasma glucose concentration
  - fasting plasma glucose concentration
  - urinalysis
- Management:
  - insulin replacement therapy
- Complications:
  - diabetic ketoacidosis (DKA)

Type 2 DM (non-insulin-dependent)
- Also called adult-onset diabetes
- Loss of insulin sensitivity
- Usually occurs in overweight people
- Commonly a family history of diabetes
- Ketoacidosis does not occur (enough insulin is produced to allow some aerobic carbohydrate metabolism)

- Symptoms:
  - polyuria
  - polydipsia
  - malaise
- Investigations:
  - plasma glucose concentration
  - fasting plasma glucose
  - urinalysis
- Management:
  - dietary control
  - metformin
- Complications:
  - microvascular: retinopathy and neuropathy
  - macrovascular: nephropathy

Cystic fibrosis-related diabetes (CFRD)

- Mostly occurs in patients with cystic fibrosis
- Managed by insulin administration

Diabetic ketoacidosis (DKA)

- Symptoms:
  - nausea
  - vomiting
  - blurred vision
  - polyuria
  - weakness
  - weight loss
- Signs:
  - tachycardia
  - confusion or coma
  - dehydration
  - hypotension
  - peripheral cyanosis
  - acetone breath
- Complications:
  - acute respiratory distress syndrome (ARDS)
  - cerebral oedema
  - thromboembolism
- Investigations:
  - urea and electrolytes
  - blood glucose concentration
  - arterial blood gases
- Management:
  - fluid replacement
  - potassium replacement
  - insulin

Diabetes insipidus
= excretion of large amounts of diluted urine
- Causes:
  - idiopathic
  - lesion in hypothalamus
  - craniopharyngioma
  - tumour metastases
  - bacterial infection (meningitis)
  - head trauma
  - drug induced
  - renal disease
- Symptoms:
  - dehydration
  - polydipsia
  - polyuria
- Investigations:
  - water deprivation test
  - blood and urine tests
- Management:
  - vasopressin

Multiple endocrine neoplasia
= inherited predisposition to develop multiple endocrine tumours (autosomal dominant condition)
- Multiple endocrine neoplasia type 1 (MEN 1)
  - tumours in parathyroid gland, pancreas and anterior pituitary gland
  - usually multiple tumours in pancreas
- Multiple endocrine neoplasia type 2 (MEN 2)
  - tumours in thyroid (medullary carcinoma), phaeochromocytoma, parathyroid (2A only) and neurofibroma (2B only)

Phaeochromocytoma
- Tumour of adrenal medulla (chromaffin cells) that produces catecholamines
- Production of noradrenaline exceeds production of adrenaline
- Rule of 10's: 10% bilateral, 10% malignant and 10% extra-adrenal
- Risk factors:
  - MEN 2
  - family history
- Symptoms:
  - headache
  - palpitations
  - sweating
  - tachycardia
  - abdominal pain
  - vomiting
  - constipation

- Signs:
  - HT
- Investigations:
  - blood tests (hyperglycaemia)
  - urinary VMA and catecholamine levels
  - CT
  - MRI
- Management:
  - surgical resection

Cushing's syndrome

- Excessive cortisol production
- More common in females
- Causes:
  - (a) prescribed prednisolone:
    - iatrogenic
    - most common cause
  - (b) adrenal adenoma/carcinoma:
    - hypersecretion of cortisol
  - (c) Cushing's disease:
    - = pituitary adenoma
    - release of ACTH
  - (d) ectopic ACTH-releasing tumour (lungs, pancreas and kidney)
- Symptoms:
  - insomnia
  - cataracts
  - bruising easily
  - muscle weakness
  - peptic ulcer
  - striae
  - polydipsia
  - menstrual disturbance
- Signs:
  - psychosis
  - osteoporosis
  - hirsutism
  - HT
  - truncal obesity
  - 'moon face'
  - 'buffalo hump' (due to increased insulin release → redistribution of fat stores to face, neck and U. trunk)
  - wasting of proximal thigh muscles
- Investigations:
  - urinary and blood cortisol levels
  - diurnal plasma cortisol levels
  - low-dose dexamethasone suppression test (normally gives negative

feedback to ACTH secretion, but in Cushing's syndrome cortisol secretion is not suppressed)
- high-dose dexamethasone suppression test
- Management:
  - metyrapone
  - trans-sphenoidal adrenalectomy (Cushing's disease)
  - adrenalectomy (adrenal adenoma)
  - tumour removal (ectopic ACTH-releasing tumour)

Nelson's syndrome
- Occurs after bilateral adrenalectomy
- Characteristic pituitary adenoma and high ACTH levels
- Signs:
  - pigmentation
- Management:
  - surgical resection of pituitary gland
  - radiotherapy

Adrenal insufficiency
- Inadequate secretion of cortisol and aldosterone
- Causes:
  (a) primary (increased levels of ACTH):
    - autoimmune
    - TB
  (b) secondary (reduced levels of ACTH):
    - pituitary disease
- Symptoms:
  - fatigue
  - hypotension

Addison's disease
- Acute adrenal insufficiency due to destruction of adrenal cortex
- Symptoms:
  - pigmentation
  - nausea
  - vomiting
  - muscle weakness
  - joint pain
  - weight loss
  - syncope
- Signs:
  - postural hypotension
  - hyperkalaemia
  - hyponatraemia
  - dehydration (due to low plasma sodium levels)
  - dizziness

  - hyperpigmentation of lips
- Investigations:
  - blood tests (plasma ACTH, high potassium, low sodium)
  - short ACTH stimulation test
  - AXR
  - CT scan of adrenal glands
- Management:
  - replacement of glucocorticoid and mineralocorticoid
- Addisonian crisis:
  - give IV fluids
  - hydrocortisone

Conn's syndrome
- Hyperaldosteronism due to production of large amounts of aldosterone
- Causes:
  - adrenal adenoma
  - bilateral adrenal hyperplasia
- Signs:
  - HT
  - hypokalaemia
  - normal or low renin levels in plasma
  - raised aldosterone levels
- Symptoms:
  - polyuria
  - lethargy
- Investigations:
  - blood tests (plasma aldosterone and renin)
  - 24-hour urinary aldosterone
  - CT scan
- Management: spironolactone pre-operatively → surgical resection (adrenalectomy)

10

Head and neck

- **External occipital protuberance**
  - attaches trapezius, sternoclcidomastoid muscle and ligamentum nuchae
  - frontal bone + parietal bones + temporal bones + sphenoid bone + occipital bone + ethmoid bone
- Metopic suture is found between frontal bones
  Lamboid suture is found between parietal and occipital bones
  Coronal suture is found between frontal and parietal bones
  Sagittal suture is found between R. and L. parietal bones
- Bregma = intersection between coronal sutures and sagittal suture (remnant of ant. fontanelle)
- Lambda = intersection between sagittal suture and lambdoid sutures
- **Cranium**
  = skull minus mandible
  - (from outermost to innermost layer) pericranium → outer table → diploe → inner table→ endocranium
- **Calvaria**
  = upper part of cranium containing the brain
  - frontal bone
  - ethmoid bone
  - sphenoid bone
  - occipital bone
  - temporal bones
  - parietal bones
- **Facial skeleton**
  = lower part of cranium
  - zygomatic bones
  - nasal bones
  - lacrimal bones

- maxillae
- inf. nasal conchae
- vomer
- **Ant. cranial fossa**
  - frontal, ethmoid and sphenoid bones (lesser wing)
  - foramen caecum for emissary veins to sup. sagittal sinus
  - crista galli of ethmoid bone: site of ant. attachments of falx cerebri
  - cribriform plates on either side of crista galli (olfactory nerves pass through)
  - contents: frontal lobes of brain
- **Middle cranial fossa**
  - sphenoid (greater wing and body) and temporal bones (petrous and squamous temporal)
  - sella turcica
    - (i) pituitary gland lies in it, bounded ant. by tuberculum sellae and post. by dorsum sellae
    - (ii) covered by diaphragma sellae
  - carotid groove
  - foramen for cranial n. and blood v.
  - (a) Optic canal
    - CNII, ophthalmic a. and central v. of retina
  - (b) Superior orbital fissure
    - CNIII, CNIV, ophthalmic division of CNV, VI
  - (c) Foramen rotundum
    - maxillary division of CNV
    - communicates with pterygopalatine fossa
  - (d) Foramen ovale
    - mandibular division of CNV
    - communicates with infratemporal fossa
  - (e) Foramen lacerum
    - int. carotid a.
    - between petrous temporal bone and sphenoid bone
  - (f) Foramen spinosum
    - middle meningeal a.
    - communicates with infratemporal fossa
    - fracture: Battle's sign
    - contents: temporal lobes
- **Posterior cranial fossa**
  - occipital and petrous temporal bones
  - foramen
  - (a) Foramen magnum
    - bounded laterally by occipital condyles
    - spinal root of CNXI, vertebral arteries and medulla oblongata
    - communicates with spinal cord
  - (b) Hypoglossal canal
    - hypoglossal n.

(c) Jugular foramen
  - between petrous temporal bone and occipital bone
  - IJV, CNIX + CNX + CNXI, sigmoid sinus
(d) Internal acoustic meatus
  - CN VII + CNVIII, labyrinthine a.
  - communicates with middle ear
  - contents: cerebellum, brainstem
- Emissary foraminas in skull transmit scalp veins to venous sinuses
- Incisive fossa transmits nasopalatine n., and sphenopalatine a. + v.
- **Pterion**
  - 4 cm above zygomatic arch
  - overlies ant. branch of middle meningeal a.
  - injury leads to extradural haematoma
- **Walls of orbit**
  - roof = orbital plate of frontal bone
  - lateral wall = zygomatic bone + zygomatic process of sphenoid bone
  - floor = maxilla + zygomatic bone
  - medial wall = ethmoid + lacrimal + sphenoid + frontal bones
- **Superior orbital fissure**
  - communication between orbit and middle cranial fossa
  - lies between greater and lesser wings of sphenoid bone
  - structures passing through: CNIII, IV, V_1, VI, ophthalmic veins
- **Inferior orbital fissure**
  - communicates with infratemporal fossa and pterygopalatine fossa
  - structures passing through: zygomatic n.
- **Supraorbital notch**
  - structures passing through: supraorbital n., supraorbital a. + v.
- **Infraorbital notch**
  - structures passing through: infraorbital n., infraorbital a. + v.
- **Zygomaticofacial foramen**
  - structures passing through: zygomaticofacial n.
- **Temporal bone**
  = squamous bone + tympanic bone + mastoid process + petrous temporal bone + zygomatic process
- **Pterion**
  - ant. branch of middle meningeal a. (from maxillary a.)
- **Temporal fossa**
  - limited laterally by temporal fascia
  - limited anteriorly by frontal process of zygomatic bone and zygomatic process of frontal bone
  - contains temporalis, zygomaticotemporal n. and middle temporal a.
- **Pterygomaxillary fissure**
  = door to pterygopalatine fossa
- **Pterygopalatine fossa**
  - contents: CNV_2 + maxillary a.
  - communicates laterally with infratemporal fossa through

pterygomaxillary fissure
- communicates medially with nasal cavity through sphenopalatine foramen
- communicates superiorly with skull through foramen rotundum
- communicates anteriorly with orbit through inferior orbital fissure
- **Infratemporal fossa**
  - lies deep to ramus of mandible
  - lies below inferior temporal line
  - lies medial to ramus of mandible
  - lies lateral to wall of pharynx
  - leads medially to pterygopalatine fossa $\rightarrow$ sphenopalatine foramen $\rightarrow$ nasal cavity
  - communicates with temporal fossa through gap between zygomatic arch and medial skull
  - contents: sphenomandibular ligament, med. + lat. pterygoid muscles + maxillary a. + CNV_3 + chorda tympani + lesser petrosal n. + pterygoid venous plexus
- **Layers of scalp** (from outermost to innermost) (can be remembered by the acronym SCALP):
  - **S**kin
  - **C**onnective tissue
  - occipitofrontalis + **A**poneurosis
  - **L**oose areolar tissue
  - **P**ericranium
- **Arterial SS of scalp**
  - supraorbital + supratrochlear a. (from ophthalmic a. of int. carotid a.)
  - superficial temporal a. (from ext. carotid a.)
  - post. auricular a. (from ext. carotid a.) SS scalp above and behind auricle
  - occipital a. (from ext. carotid a.) SS back of scalp
- **Venous drainage of scalp**
  - supratrochlear v. + supraorbital v. $\rightarrow$ facial v.
  - superficial temporal v. + maxillary v. $\rightarrow$ retromandibular v. $\rightarrow$ ext. jugular v.
  - occipital v. $\rightarrow$ IJV
- **Lymphatic drainage of scalp**
  - ant. scalp: submandibular nodes
  - lat. scalp: parotid nodes
  - behind ear: mastoid nodes
  - back of scalp: occipital nodes
- Subaponeurotic space is limited anteriorly and posteriorly by origins of occipitofrontalis, and laterally by temporal fascia
- **Pharyngeal arch**
  - core mesenchymal tissue enclosed by surface ectoderm
  - contain their own cranial n., arterial supply and muscular components
  - externally separated by grooves, and internally separated by pouches
  - arch I (SS m. of mastication, tensor tympani) (nerve SS: CNV_2, V_3)

- arch II (SS m. of facial expression, stapedius) (nerve SS: CNVII)
- arch III (SS stylopharyngeus) (nerve SS: CNIX)
- arch IV (SS cricothyroid + intrinsic m. of soft palate except tensor veli palatini) (nerve SS: CNX SLN)
- arch VI (SS intrinsic m. of larynx except cricothyroid m.) (nerve SS: CNX RLN)
- first pharyngeal groove becomes external ear canal
- first pharyngeal pouch (tympanic cavity), second pharyngeal pouch (tonsils), third pharyngeal pouch (thymus), fourth pharyngeal pouch (parathyroid glands)
- **Internal carotid a.**
  - begins at level of U. border of thyroid cartilage (C3/4)
  - no branches in neck
  - enters skull through carotid canal
  - passes into cavernous sinus
  - gives off ophthalmic a.
  - terminal branches = ant. cerebral a. + middle cerebral a.
- **External carotid a.**
  - begins at level of U. border of thyroid cartilage (C3/4)
  - runs anterior and lateral to internal carotid a.
  - runs deep to posterior belly of digastric m.
  - terminal branches = superficial temporal a. + maxillary a.
- **Branches of external carotid a.**
  - (a) Ant. branches
    - superior thyroid a.
    - lingual a.
    - facial a.
  - (b) Post. branches
    - occipital a.
    - post. auricular a.
  - (c) Medial branch
    - ascending pharyngeal a.
- **Arterial SS of face**
  - (a) Facial a.
    - from ext. carotid a.
    - follows a tortuous course from the ant. edge of the masseter, along the side of the nose to the medial angle of the eye
    - terminates as angular a.
    - pulse can be felt inf. to mandible ant. to masseter
    - branches = submental a., sup. + inf. labial a., and lat. nasal a.
  - (b) Superficial temporal a.
    - one of the terminal branches of ext. carotid a.
  - (c) Transverse facial a.
    - branch of superficial temporal a.
  - (d) Supraorbital a. + supratrochlear a.
    - branches of ophthalmic a. (from int. carotid a.)

- **Venous drainage of face**
  - facial v. formed by supraorbital and supratrochlear v.
  - connected to superior ophthalmic v. → connected to cavernous sinus → path for spreading infection from face to cavernous sinus
- **Larynx**
  - epiglottis + thyroid cartilage + cricoid cartilage + arytenoid cartilage
  - arterial SS:
    - (i) sup. laryngeal a. (from sup. thyroid a.)
    - (ii) inf. laryngeal a. (from inf. thyroid a.)
  - nerve SS:
    - (i) sup. laryngeal n. (motor SS cricothyroid + inf. constrictor m.; sensory SS mucosa of false vocal folds, piriform sinuses)
    - (ii) RLN (motor SS all intrinsic m. of larynx; sensory SS mucosa of true vocal folds)
- **Arytenoid cartilages**
  - pyramidal cartilages forming part of larynx
  - attach vocal cords
  - sit on U. border of lamina of cricoid cartilage
- **Cuneiform cartilages**
  - yellow elastic cartilage
  - in aryepiglottic fold
- **Corniculate cartilages**
  - yellow elastic cartilage
  - in base of aryepiglottic fold
  - on apex of arytenoid cartilages
- **Quadrangular membrane**
  - between epiglottis and arytenoid
  - sup. margin: aryepiglottic fold
  - inf. margin: vestibular ligament (false vocal cord)
- **Cricoarytenoid joints (act on vocal process)**
  - (a) Post. cricoarytenoid:
    - from back of cricoid cartilage → muscular process of arytenoid cartilage
    - abduct vocal ligament
  - (b) Lat. cricoarytenoid:
    - from U. border of cricoid cartilage → muscular process of arytenoid cartilage
    - adduct vocal ligament
  - (c) Transverse arytenoid:
    - only unpaired structure
    - adduct vocal ligament
  - (d) Oblique arytenoid:
    - from muscular process of arytenoid → apex of opposite arytenoid
    - adduct vocal ligament
- **Cricothyroid membrane**

- sup. margin attached to post. thyroid cartilage + vocal process of arytenoid cartilage
- sup. margin thickened to form vocal ligament
- inf. margin = cricoid cartilage
- **Attachments of vocal ligaments (true vocal folds)**
  - post. thyroid cartilage
  - vocal processes of arytenoid cartilages
- **Hyoid bone**
  - U-shaped
  - body + greater horn + lesser horn
  - vertebral level: C3
- **Attachments of hyoid bone**
  - inf.: larynx
  - sup.: floor of oral cavity
  - post.: pharynx
- **Boundaries of anterior triangle of neck**
  - ant. border of sternocleidomastoid
  - midline of neck
  - lower border of mandible
- **Roof of ant. triangle = platysma + fascia**
  Floor of ant. triangle = mylohyoid + hyoglossus + infrahyoid + pharynx constrictors
- **Boundaries of posterior triangle of neck**
  - post. border of sternocleidomastoid
  - middle third of clavicle
  - ant. border of trapezius
- **Contents of posterior triangle of neck**
  - third part of subclavian a.
  - cutaneous branches of cervical plexus
  - brachial plexus trunks
  - inf. belly of omohyoid
  - spinal part of accessory n.
  - cervical lymph nodes
- **Muscles forming floor of post. triangle of neck**
  - post. scalenus
  - middle scalenus
  - levator scapulae
  - splenius capitis
- **Columns of the neck**
  - bony muscular column (enclosed by prevert. fascia)
  - visceral column (enclosed by pretracheal fascia)
  - neurovascular bundles (surrounded by carotid sheath)
  - whole neck (enclosed by deep investing fascia)
- **Attachments for sternocleidomastoid muscle**
  - origin: manubrium + medial third of clavicle
  - insertion: mastoid process of temporal bone + sup. nuchal line

- nerve SS: spinal root of accessory n. (CNXI)
- function: rotate head to ipsilat. side (act alone) + protrude head and assist in forced inspiration (act together)
- **Attachments for platysma muscle**
  - origin: deep fascia over pectoralis major
  - insertion: inf. border of mandible + angle of mouth
  - nerve SS: cervical branch of facial n. (CNVII)
  - function: pull corners of mouth down
- **Suprahyoid muscles**
  - mylohyoid muscle
  - digastric muscle
  - geniohyoid muscle
  - stylohyoid muscle
- **Attachments of mylohyoid muscle**
  - origin: mylohyoid line in mandible
  - insertion: median raphe and hyoid bone
  - nerve SS: CNV_3
  - function: elevate hyoid bone
- **Attachments of digastric muscle**
  - origin: (ant. belly) mandible
    (post. belly) temporal bone
  - insertion: bellies connected by a tendon
  - nerve SS: (ant. belly) CNV_3
    (post. belly) CNVII
- **Attachments of geniohyoid muscle**
  - origin: genial tubercle of mandible
  - insertion: hyoid bone
  - nerve SS: C1
  - function: elevate hyoid bone
- **Attachments of stylohyoid muscle**
  - origin: styloid process
  - insertion: hyoid bone
  - nerve SS: CNVII
  - function: elevate hyoid bone
- **Infrahyoid strap muscles**
  - sternohyoid muscle
  - omohyoid muscle
  - sternothyroid muscle
  - thyrohyoid muscle
- **Attachments of sternohyoid muscle**
  - origin: manubrium
  - insertion: hyoid bone
  - nerve SS: ansa cervicalis C1–3
  - function: depress hyoid bone
- **Attachments of omohyoid muscle**
  - origin: hyoid bone

- insertion: scapula
- nerve SS: ansa cervicalis C1–3
- function: depress hyoid bone
- **Attachments of sternothyroid muscle**
  - origin: manubrium
  - insertion: thyroid cartilage
  - nerve SS: ansa cervicalis C1–3
  - function: depress larynx
- **Attachments of thyrohyoid muscle**
  - origin: thyroid cartilage
  - insertion: hyoid bone
  - nerve SS: CNXII
  - function: depress hyoid bone
- Sup. temporal v. + maxillary v. (join in parotid gland) = retro-mandibular v.
- **Sup. veins of neck: EJV and AJV**
  - (a) EJV:
    - formed post. to angle of mandible (post. auricular v. and post. retromandibular v. join)
    - descend across sternocleidomastoid muscle post. to subclavian v.
  - (b) AJV:
    - begin as small v. below chin, come together at hyoid bone → descend on midline of neck → pierce investing layer of cervical fascia to enter subclavian v.
- **Cervical sympathetic ganglia in neck**
  - superior cervical ganglion (at level C2,3)
  - middle cervical ganglion (at level C6)
  - inferior cervical ganglion (at level T1)
- **Cranial nerves**
  (*see* Table 10.1)
- **Optic n.**
  - surrounded by layers of meninges + subarachnoid space
  - pierced by central a. + v. of retina
- **Oculomotor n.**
  - superior division: SS sup. rectus + levator palpebrae superioris
  - inferior division: SS inf. rectus + medial rectus + inf. oblique
  - gives parasym. fibres to ciliary ganglion
- **Edinger–Westphal nucleus**
  - on post. aspect of oculomotor nucleus in midbrain
  - fibres pass to ciliary ganglion through inferior division of CNIII
  - causes contraction of ciliary m. and constriction of pupils
- **Pathway for pupillary light reflex**
  - retina → optic n. → pretectal n. in midbrain → Edinger–Westphal nucleus → oculomotor n. → ciliary ganglion → constrictor pupillae
- Trochlear n. = only cranial n. arising from post. brainstem
- Abducens n. = cranial n. with longest intracranial course
  - vulnerable to increased ICP

Table 10.1 Properties of cranial nerves I–XII

Cranial nerve	Type of nerve fibre	Function	Foramen in skull	Course	Lesion
I (olfactory)	Sensory	Smell	Cribriform plate of ethmoid	Axons from olfactory bulb form olfactory tract → cortex	Anosmia (mostly caused by U. resp. tract infections such as rhinitis/head injury)
II (optic)	Sensory	Vision	Optic canal	Ganglion cells → optic n. → optic canal → decussate to form optic chiasma → optic tract (medial half cross midline)	Visual acuity affected, loss of pupillary constriction
III (oculomotor)	Motor	Motor SS to levator palpebrae superioris + medial + superior + inferior rectus + inferior oblique; raise U. eyelid; turn cornea upwards, downwards and medially; constricts pupil; accommodation	Superior orbital fissure	Arises from ant. midbrain oculomotor nucleus + Edinger–Westphal nucleus; enters orbit between two heads of lat. rectus within fibrous ring; inf. division gives branch with preganglionic parasympathetic n. to ciliary ganglion → SS ciliary muscles (accommodation), sphincter pupillae (constriction)	Lateral squint (unopposed action of lateral rectus + superior oblique), dilated pupil, ptosis (paralysis of levator palpebrae superioris), loss of light reflex
IV (trochlear)	Motor	Motor SS to superior oblique; turn cornea downward and laterally	Superior orbital fissure	From post. brainstem (trochlear nucleus) → runs to ant. midbrain → lat. wall of cavernous sinus; tendon passes through trochlea	Trouble looking down when walking downstairs

Cranial nerve	Type of nerve fibre	Function	Foramen in skull	Course	Lesion
V₁ (trigeminal, ophthalmic division)	Sensory	Supply cornea, skin of forehead, eyelids, scalp, nasal cavity mucous membranes	Superior orbital fissure	Arises from lat. aspect of pons → trigeminal ganglion on temporal bone → divides into three divisions	
V₂ (maxillary division)	Sensory	Supply skin over maxilla, temple, U. jaw, nose, palate	Foramen rotundum		
V₃ (mandibular division)	Motor, sensory	Motor SS to muscles of mastication, mylohyoid, ant. belly of digastric, tensor veli palatini, tensor tympani; sensory SS to skin over cheek, lower jaw, mouth, ant. tongue	Foramen ovale		
VI (abducens)	Motor	Motor SS to lateral rectus; turns cornea laterally	Superior orbital fissure	From abducens nucleus → runs between pons and medulla near midline; pierces dura at clivus → grooves tip of petrous bone → cavernous sinus → sup. orbital fissure within fibrous ring between heads of lat. rectus	Diplopia

(continued)

Table 10.1 Properties of cranial nerves I–XII (*continued*)

Cranial nerve	Type of nerve fibre	Function	Foramen in skull	Course	Lesion
VII (facial)	Motor, sensory, secretomotor	Motor SS to muscles of facial expression, stapedius muscle, post. belly of digastric, stylohyoid, platysma; taste from ant. two-thirds of tongue; secretomotor to submandibular + sublingual salivary glands, lacrimal glands, glands of nose; sensory SS from auricle	Internal acoustic meatus, stylomastoid foramen	Arises from cerebellopontine angle; facial canal in petrous temporal bone → stylomastoid foramen; greater petrosal n. joins deep petrosal n.; chorda tympani joins lingual n., gives taste to ant. two-thirds of tongue and gives parasympathetic SS to submandibular and sublingual salivary glands, lacrimal glands	Bell's palsy
VIII (vestibulocochlear)	Sensory	Receives sensory impulses from utricle, saccule, semicircular canals and organ of Corti	Internal acoustic meatus	Cerebellopontine angle → around inf. cerebellar peduncle → int. acoustic meatus	Unilateral deafness, tinnitus
IX (glossopharyngeal)	Motor, sensory, secretomotor	Motor SS to stylopharyngeus; sensory from post. tongue, U. pharynx; taste from post. third of tongue, afferent fibres from carotid sinus + body; secretomotor to parotid salivary gland (through otic ganglion)	Jugular foramen	From nucleus ambiguus (motor)/ nucleus of solitary tract (sensory)/inf. salivatory nucleus (parasym.) → between olive, inf. cerebellar peduncle → jugular foramen ant. to CNX, CNXI → sup. + inf. ganglia → down + lat. between int. carotid a. and jugular v. → between ext. + int. carotid a. along lat. border of stylopharyngeus	Loss of taste + sensation from post. third of tongue

Cranial nerve	Type of nerve fibre	Function	Foramen in skull	Course	Lesion
X (vagus)	Motor, sensory, parasympathetic	Motor SS to palatoglossus, muscles of larynx + pharynx except stylopharyngeus and tensor veli palatini; sensory from external acoustic meatus, heart, blood vessels, lungs, abdominal viscera, aortic bodies; parasympathetic to heart, lungs, abdominal viscera	Jugular foramen	From medulla → carotid sheath (medial to IJV)	Deviation of uvula to normal side; paralysis of vocal cord
XI (accessory)	Motor	(cranial root) Motor SS to muscles of soft palate (except tensor veli palatini), pharynx (except stylopharyngeus), larynx (except cricothyroid); (spinal root) motor SS to sternocleidomastoid, trapezius	Jugular foramen	From nucleus ambiguus (cranial root)/ant. horns of C1–6 (spinal root); goes through foramen magnum (spinal root)	Paresis of sternocleidomastoid + trapezius
XII (hypoglossal)	Motor	Motor SS to muscles of tongue (except palatoglossus)	Hypoglossal canal	From hypoglossal nucleus in medulla; rootlets lie between pyramid and olive of medulla	Protruded tongue deviates to side of lesion

- Glossopharyngeal n. + vagus n. + accessory n. arise from rootlets lateral to olive in medulla
- Accessory n. vulnerable to damage during neck surgery
- Hypoglossal n. passes over loop on lingual a. → lies below submandibular duct
- **Branches of ophthalmic division of trigeminal n. (CNV$_1$)**
  - SS skin of forehead, U. eyelid and lateral aspect of nose
    - (a) Frontal n.
      - supraorbital n.
      - supratrochlear n.
    - (b) Lacrimal n. (receives parasympathetic fibres from pterygopalatine ganglion)
    - (c) Nasociliary n.
      - long ciliary n. (contains sym. fibres)
      - short ciliary n. (contains parasym. fibres)
      - ant. ethmoidal n.
- **Branches of maxillary division of trigeminal n. (CNV$_2$)**
  - SS skin of L. eyelid, cheeks and U. lip
    - (a) Infra-orbital n.
    - (b) Zygomatic n.
      - zygomaticofacial n.
      - zygomaticotemporal n.
    - (c) Superior alveolar n.
    - (d) Greater and lesser palatine n.
- **Branches of mandibular division of trigeminal n. (CNV$_3$)**
  - SS skin of L. lip and temporal region
    - (a) Buccal n.
    - (b) Lingual n.
    - (c) Inferior alveolar n.
    - (d) Auriculotemporal n.
- **Lesion of trigeminal n.**
  - anaesthesia of face and scalp
  - paralysis of muscles of mastication
- **Motor branches of facial n. emerge from ant. aspect of parotid gland**
  - temporal branch: runs upwards to orbit
  - zygomatic branch: runs horizontally, crossing zygomatic arch
  - buccal branch: runs anteriorly to nose and U. lip
  - mandibular branch: runs along lower margin of mandible
  - cervical branch: runs below inf. border of parotid gland
- **Facial v.**
  - connected with ophthalmic veins and pterygoid venous plexus
  - may spread superficial infection into cranium
- **Dural venous sinuses**
  - receive venous drainage from cerebral veins
  - drain to IJV
    - (a) Sup. sagittal sinus

      – begins at foramen cecum where it receives blood from emissary
       vein of foramen cecum → drains into R. transverse sinus
- (b) Inf. sagittal sinus
  - receives cerebral v.
  - joins great cerebral v. → straight sinus
- (c) Straight sinus
  - drains into L. transverse sinus → confluence of sinuses
- (d) Occipital sinus
  - drains to confluence of sinuses
- (e) Confluence of sinuses
  - drains to transverse sinuses
- (f) Transverse sinuses
  - drains to sigmoid sinuses → drains into IJV
- (g) Superior petrosal sinus
  - receives cavernous sinus
  - drains to transverse sinus → sigmoid sinus
- (h) Inferior petrosal sinus
  - receives cavernous sinus
  - drains to IJV
- (i) Cavernous sinus
  - drains blood from pterygoid plexus of veins + inf. and sup. ophthalmic veins + middle and inf. cerebral veins → petrosal sinuses

- **Structures embedded in cavernous sinus**
  - lateral wall: CNV1 + CNV2, CNIII, CNIV
  - pass through centre: CNVI, int. carotid artery and sympathetic plexus
- **Arachnoid granulations**
  - arachnoid mater that protrude into sup. sagittal sinus
  - transport CSF produced by the choroid plexuses into the circulation
- **Course of int. cartotid a.**
  - carotid canal → cavernous sinus → terminate as ant. + middle cerebral a.
- **Muscles of facial expression**
  - frontalis
  - orbicularis oculi
  - orbicularis oris
  - buccinator
- **Attachments of occipitofrontalis muscle**
  - origin (frontal belly): skin around eyebrow
  - origin (occipital belly): sup. nuchal line of occipital bone + mastoid process of temporal bone
  - epicranial aponeurosis connects frontal bellies with occipital bellies
  - insertion: epicranial aponeurosis
  - nerve SS (frontal belly): temporal branch of facial n. (CNVII)
  - nerve SS (occipital belly): post. auricular branch of facial n. (CNVII)
  - function: raises eyebrows
- **Attachments of orbicularis oculi muscle**

- origin (palpebral part): medial palpebral ligament
- origin (orbital part): nasal part of frontal bone + frontal process of maxilla
- insertion (palpebral part): lat. palpebral raphe
- insertion (orbital part): circle around orbit
- nerve SS: zygomatic branch of facial n. (CNVII)
- function: closes eyelids gently (palpebral part) or forcefully (orbital part)
- **Attachments of orbicularis oris muscle**
  - origin: maxilla + mandible
  - insertion: circles around mouth
  - nerve SS: buccal branch of facial n. (CNVII)
  - function: closes and protrudes lips; compresses distended cheeks
- **Attachments of buccinator muscle**
  - origin: post. parts of maxilla + mandible; pterygomandibular raphe
  - insertion: orbicularis oris
  - nerve SS: buccal branch of facial n. (CNVII)
  - function: compresses cheeks inwards against teeth
- **Muscles of mastication**
  - masseter
  - temporalis
  - lat. pterygoid
  - med. pterygoid
- **Attachments of masseter muscle**
  - origin: zygomatic arch + maxillary process of zygomatic bone
  - insertion: lat. ramus of mandible
  - nerve SS: mandibular n. (CNV$_3$)
  - function: elevates mandible
- **Attachments of temporalis muscle**
  - origin: temporal fossa + fascia
  - insertion: coronoid process of mandible + ramus of mandible
  - nerve SS: mandibular n. (CNV$_3$)
  - function (anterior fibres): elevates mandible
  - function (posterior fibres): retracts mandible
- **Attachments of lat. pterygoid muscle**
  - origin (U. head): infratemporal surface of temporal bone (greater wing of sphenoid)
  - origin (L. head): lat. surface of lat. pterygoid plate
  - insertion: neck of mandible
  - nerve SS: n. to lat. pterygoid (ant. division of mandibular n. CNV$_3$)
  - function: protract and depress and move mandible from side to side
- **Attachments of med. pterygoid muscle**
  - origin (deep head): medial surface of lat. pterygoid plate
  - origin (superficial head): maxilla
  - insertion: medial surface of angle of mandible
  - nerve SS: n. to medial pterygoid (mandibular n. CNV$_3$)
  - function: protract and elevate and move mandible from side to side
- **Pharynx**

- from base of skull → C6
- constrictor muscles (sup. + middle + inf. constrictors)
- longitudinal muscles (stylopharyngeus, palatopharyngeus and salpingopharyngeus)

- **Attachments of superior constrictor muscle**
  - origin: pterygoid hamulus, pterygomandibular raphe, post. part of mylohyoid line
  - insertion: pharyngeal raphe (post. pharynx)
  - nerve SS: vagus n.
  - function: propel food bolus
- **Attachments of middle constrictor muscle**
  - origin: hyoid bone
  - insertion: pharyngeal raphe (post. pharynx)
  - nerve SS: vagus n.
  - function: propel food bolus
- **Attachments of inferior constrictor muscle**
  - origin: thyroid + cricoid cartilage
  - insertion: pharyngeal raphe (post. pharynx)
  - nerve SS: vagus n.
  - function: propel food bolus
- **Attachments of stylopharyngeus muscle**
  - origin: styloid process
  - insertion: posterolateral thyroid cartilage
  - nerve SS: glossopharyngeal n. (CNIX)
  - function: elevate larynx and pharynx
- **Attachments of palatopharyngeus muscle**
  - origin: hard palate
  - insertion: U. border of thyroid cartilage
  - nerve SS: vagus n. (CNX)
  - function: elevate larynx and pharynx
- **Attachments of salpingopharyngeus muscle**
  - origin: inf. part of Eustachian tube
  - insertion: U. border of thyroid cartilage
  - nerve SS: vagus n. (CNX)
  - function: elevate larynx and pharynx
- **Nasopharynx**
  - from base of skull to soft palate
  - continuous with nasal cavity through choanae
  - nasopharyngeal tonsil (adenoids)
  - opening of Eustachian tube (can spread infection from nasopharynx to middle ear)
- **Oropharynx**
  - from soft palate to epiglottis
  - continuous with oral cavity through oropharyngeal isthmus
  - palatine tonsils (lie between palatoglossal arch and palatopharyngeal arch)

- arterial SS of tonsils: tonsillar branch of facial a.
- venous drainage of tonsils: paratonsillar v.
- lymphatic drainage of tonsils: jugulodigastric node
- Roof of oral cavity = hard palate + soft palate
- **Hard palate**
  - palatine plate of maxilla + horizontal plate of palatine bone
- **Sensory SS of roof of oral cavity**
  - ant.: greater palatine n. + nasopalatine n. (branches of CNV$_2$)
  - post.: glossopharyngeal n. (CNIX)
- **Muscles of soft palate**
  - tensor veli palatini
  - levator veli palatini
  - palatoglossus
  - palatopharyngeus
- **Innervation of muscles of soft palate**
  - CNX (all except tensor veli palatini)
  - CNV$_3$ (tensor veli palatini)

Common pathologies

Trigeminal neuropathy
- Mostly caused by herpes simplex virus
- Unilateral sensory loss involving the face

Bell's palsy
- Acute onset of unilateral facial weakness
- Most common causes:
  - viral (herpes → Ramsay Hunt syndrome)
  - brainstem tumour
- Symptoms:
  - paralysis of U. + L. facial muscles (forehead wrinkles disappear, dry eye, facial drooping, drooling, altered sense of taste)
  - hyperacusis (stapedius)
  - reduced secretion of tears and saliva
  - loss of taste in ant. two-thirds of tongue
- Test: wrinkle forehead, close eyes tightly
- Management:
  - lubricating ointment for dry eyes

Parkinson's disease
- Neurodegenerative disease
- Usual age of onset: 40–70 years
- Most common cause: progressive degeneration of dopaminergic neurons in substantia nigra (after stroke or repeated head trauma, or drug induced)
- Characteristic lesion: Lewy bodies

- Symptoms:
  - akinesia
  - bradykinesia (blank expressionless face, shuffling gait, and loss of arm swing)
  - cogwheel rigidity
  - resting tremor (4–6 Hz)
  - flexed posture
  - dysphagia
- Management:
  - physiotherapy
  - L-dopa with decarboxylase inhibitors
  - anticholinergics (for treating tremors)
  - dopamine-receptor (D_2) agonists (bromocriptine)
  - monoamine oxidase B inhibitors, COMT inhibitors

Dementia
= progressive deterioration in cognitive functions
- Causes:
  - Alzheimer's disease
  - dementia with Lewy bodies
  - Parkinson's disease
  - vitamin B_{12} deficiency
  - repeated trauma (e.g. in boxers)
  - cerebrovascular disease
  - subdural haematoma
  - hypothyroidism
  - infections
  - uraemia
  - alcohol
- Investigations:
  - blood tests
  - CXR
  - EEG
  - CT scan

Alzheimer's disease
- Neurodegenerative disease
- Common cause of dementia
- Pathological characteristics: amyloid plaques and neurofibrillary tangles
- Symptoms:
  - recent memory loss
  - spatial disorientation
  - aphasia
  - apraxia
  - agnosia (inability to recognise places or people)
  - change in personality (aggressive)

- Investigations: MRI of brain
- Management: acetylcholinesterase (rivastigmine)

Stroke

= acute onset of focal CNS signs due to vascular causes
- Mostly affects middle cerebral artery
- Risk factors:
  - genetics
  - age
  - gender (male)
  - family history
  - obesity
  - hyperlipidaemia
  - DM
  - HT
  - smoking
  - alcohol abuse
  - heart disease (heart failure, endocarditis)
  - atrial fibrillation
  - previous MI
  - oral contraceptive pill
- Causes:
  - (a) cerebral infarction:
    - most common
    - embolism from clots
  - (b) intracerebral haemorrhage:
    - represents around 10% of cases
  - (c) subarachnoid haemorrhage
- Signs:
  - (a) cerebral hemisphere:
    - contralateral hemiplagia and sensory loss, UMN signs, aphasia (if dominant lobe affected)
  - (b) lacunar infarcts (small hole-like infarcts around the basal ganglia, internal capsule, thalamus and pons):
    - pure sensory, motor or mixed ataxia
  - (c) brainstem infarcts:
    - affect CN 5, 7, 9 and 10 nuclei, corticospinal tracts and spinothalamic tracts
    - facial numbness, weakness, dysphagia, dysarthria, quadriplegia and sensory loss
  - (d) cerebellum infarcts:
    - ataxia, vertigo
    - murmurs
- Investigations:
  - CT/MRI immediately
  - carotid Doppler

- Complications:
  - cerebral oedema → increase in ICP
  - seizures
- Management:
  - thrombolysis (within 3 hours of onset + no sign of haemorrhage)
  - antiplatelet drugs, e.g. aspirin (no sign of haemorrhage)
  - heparin and warfarin (for atrial fibrillation)

Transient ischaemic attack (TIA)
= stroke with symptoms that completely resolve within 24 hours of onset
- Common cause: microemboli
- High probability of recurrence

Cerebellar lesions (occur ipsilateral to lesion)
- Causes:
  - acoustic neuroma
  - medulloblastoma
  - infarction
  - infections
  - lead poisoning
  - carbon monoxide poisoning
  - hydrocephalus
- Symptoms:
  - intention tremor (detected in finger–nose test)
  - past-pointing
  - ataxia
  - dysdiadochokinesia (inability to perform alternating movements)
  - hypotonia
  - nystagmus
  - dysarthria
  - dysmetria

11

Upper limb

- **Clavicle**
  - articulates medially with sternum
  - articulates laterally with acromion (acromioclavicular joint)
  - commonly fractured
  - weakest part = point between medial two-thirds and lateral third
- **Scapula**
  - acromion process (articulates with clavicle, provides attachment for arm and chest muscles)
  - coracoid process (provides attachment for arm and chest muscles)
  - spine (at post. aspect, attached to acromion) (at level of spinous process of T3)
  - glenoid cavity (articulates with head of humerus)
  - sup. angle at level T2; inf. angle at level T8
  - movements: protracts, retracts, elevates, depresses, medial rotation, lateral rotation
- **Attachments of biceps brachii muscle**
  - origin (long head): supraglenoid tubercle of scapula (passes through transverse humeral ligament)
  - origin (short head): coracoid process of scapula
  - insertion: bicipital tuberosity of radius
  - nerve SS: musculocutaneous n. (C5 and 6)
  - function: flex elbow, supinate forearm when elbow is flexed
- **Attachments of coracobrachialis muscle**
  - origin: coracoid process of scapula
  - insertion: middle third of medial humerus
  - nerve SS: musculocutaneous n. (C5–7)
  - function: flex and adduct arm

- **Attachments of brachialis muscle**
  - origin: ant. humerus
  - insertion: tuberosity of ulna
  - nerve SS: musculocutaneous n. (C5–7)
  - function: flex elbow
- **Attachments of triceps brachii muscle**
  - origin (long head): infraglenoid tubercle of scapula
  - origin (lateral head): U. half of post. humerus
  - origin (medial head): L. half of post. humerus
  - insertion: olecranon process of ulna
  - nerve SS: radial n. (C6–8)
  - function: stabilise shoulder joint and extend forearm
- **Attachments of supinator**
  - origin (superficial part): lat. epicondyle of humerus
  - origin (deep part): supinator crest of ulna
  - insertion: lat. surface of radius
  - nerve SS: post. interosseous n.
  - function: supinate forearm
- **Humerus**
  - head (articulates with glenoid cavity of scapula)
  - anatomical neck (proximal to greater and lesser tubercles)
  - greater and lesser tubercle (ant. aspect) (for attachment of rotator cuff muscles)
  - intertubercular groove (where tendon of biceps brachii is located)
  - surgical neck (axillary n. and post. circumflex humeral a. are closely related) (risk of injury during dislocation of shoulder/fractures in the area)
  - deltoid tuberosity (attachment for deltoid)
  - medial epicondyle (ulnar n. lies post. to it)
  - lateral epicondyle
  - trochlea (medial condyle that articulates with trochlear notch of ulna)
  - capitulum (lateral condyle that articulates with radius head)
  - coronoid fossa (ant. aspect, depression for ulna when elbow is bent)
  - olecranon fossa (post. aspect, depression for ulna when elbow is extended)
  - radial n. runs infero-laterally down post. shaft of humerus (along spiral groove)
- **Elbow joint**
  - synovial joint
  - between trochlea of humerus and trochlear notch of ulna
  - between capitulum of humerus and head of radius
  - between radial notch of ulna and radius
  - reinforced by annular ligament of radius + ulnar collateral ligament + radial collateral ligament
- **Ulna**
  - olecranon process (articulates with olecranon fossa when elbow is extended)

- – trochlear notch (articulates with trochlea of humerus)
  - – coronoid process (articulates with coronoid fossa when elbow is bent)
  - – styloid process
- **Radius**
  - – head (articulates with capitulum of humerus and radial notch of ulna)
  - – radial tuberosity (attaches tendon from biceps brachii)
  - – styloid process (more distal to styloid process of ulna)
  - – articulates with scaphoid and lunate distally
- Interosseous membrane between ulna and radius
- **Attachments of teres minor muscle**
  - – origin: lat. aspect of inf. angle of scapula (above origin of teres major)
  - – insertion: greater tubercle of humerus
  - – nerve SS: axillary n. (C5 and 6)
  - – function: laterally rotate arm, stabilise shoulder joint
- **Attachments of teres major**
  - – origin: post. surface of inf. angle of scapula
  - – insertion: medial lip of bicipital groove of humerus
  - – nerve SS: subscapular n. (C5–7)
  - – function: adduct and medially rotate arm, stabilise shoulder joint
- **Attachments of subscapularis**
  - – origin: subscapular fossa
  - – insertion: lesser tubercle of humerus
  - – nerve SS: U. + L. subscapular n. (C5 and 6)
  - – function: medially rotate arm, stabilise shoulder joint
  - – separated from shoulder joint by a large bursa
- **Attachments of supraspinatus**
  - – origin: supraspinous fossa of scapula
  - – insertion: sup. facet of greater tuberosity of humerus
  - – nerve SS: suprascapular n. (C5 and 6)
  - – function: abduct arm, stabilise shoulder joint
- **Attachments of infraspinatus**
  - – origin: infraspinous fossa of scapula
  - – insertion: middle facet of greater tuberosity of humerus
  - – nerve SS: suprascapular n. (C5 and 6)
  - – function: laterally rotate arm, stabilise shoulder joint
- **Attachments of levator scapulae**
  - – origin: post. tubercles of transverse processes of C1–4
  - – insertion: U. part of medial border of scapula
  - – nerve SS: ant. rami of C3, 4 + dorsal scapular n. (C5)
  - – function: elevate scapula
- **Rotator cuff muscles (remembered by SITS) (stabilise GH joint)**
  - – supraspinatus
  - – infraspinatus
  - – teres minor
  - – subscapularis
- **Attachments of deltoid**

- origin: lat. third of clavicle, acromion, spine of scapula
- insertion: deltoid tuberosity of humerus
- nerve SS: axillary n. (C5 and 6)
- function: abduct (middle fibres) and flex and medially rotate (ant. fibres), extend and laterally rotate (post. fibres) arm
- **Shoulder joint consists of four joints**
  - glenohumeral joint
  - sternoclavicular joint
  - acromioclavicular joint
  - scapulothoracic joint
- **Glenohumeral (GH) joint**
  - movements: flexion, extension, adduction, abduction, internal rotation, external rotation
- **Axillary a.**
  - continuation of subclavian a.
  - divided into three parts by pectoralis minor muscle
    - (a) First part (medial to pectoralis minor)
      - (i) sup. thoracic a.
    - (b) Second part (post. to pectoralis minor)
      - (i) thoraco-acromial a.
      - (ii) lat. thoracic a.
    - (c) Third part (lat. to pectoralis minor)
      - (i) subscapular a.
        - thoracodorsal a.
        - circumflex scapular a.
      - (ii) ant. circumflex humeral a.
      - (iii) post. circumflex humeral a.
- **Brachial a. (continuation of axillary a.)**
  - gives off profunda brachii a.
  - terminates as ulnar and radial a.
- **Profunda brachii a.**
  - runs in radial groove
  - passes through triangular interval with radial n.
  - anastomoses with post. circumflex humeral a. around elbow joint
- **Radial artery**
  - originates at neck of radius
  - lateral to tendon of flexor carpi radialis
  - superficial palmar branch
  - deep palmar branch
  - radial recurrent artery (around elbow joint)
- **Ulnar artery**
  - larger branch than radial artery
  - common interosseous artery (divides into ant. and post. interosseous arteries)
  - ulnar recurrent artery (around elbow joint)
- **Cephalic vein (superficial vein)**

- – pierces clavipectoral fascia
- – begins post. to styloid process of radius → lat. border of forearm → cubital fossa → lat. to biceps → groove between pectoralis major and deltoid muscle
- – drains into axillary vein
- **Boundaries of quadrangular space**
  - – med.: long head of triceps brachii
  - – sup.: inf. margin of subscapularis
  - – lat.: surgical neck of humerus
  - – inf.: sup. margin of teres major
- **Structures passing through quadrangular space**
  - – axillary n.
  - – post. circumflex humeral a. + v.
- **Boundaries of triangular space**
  - – med.: long head of triceps brachii
  - – sup.: inf. margin of subscapularis
  - – lat.: long head of triceps brachii
- **Structures passing through triangular space**
  - – circumflex scapular a. + v.
- **Boundaries of triangular interval**
  - – med.: long head of triceps brachii
  - – sup.: inf. margin of teres major
  - – lat.: shaft of humerus
- **Structures passing through triangular interval**
  - – radial n.
  - – profunda brachii a.
- **Brachial plexus**
  - – ventral rami of C5–8, T1
  - – ventral rami of C5 gives off dorsal scapular n.
  - – ventral rami of C5–7 gives off long thoracic n.
  - – ventral rami of C5 and 6 → U. trunk
  - – ventral rami of C7 → middle trunk
  - – ventral rami of C8, T1 → L. trunk
  - – U. trunk gives off suprascapular n. + n. to subclavius
  - – ant. division of U. and middle trunk → lateral cord
  - – ant. division of L. trunk → posterior cord
  - – post. division of U. + middle + L. trunk → posterior cord
  - – lateral cord gives off lateral pectoral n.; terminates as musculocutaneous n. + lat. root of median n.
  - – medial cord gives off medial pectoral n.; terminates as ulnar n. + med. root of median n.
  - – posterior cord gives off U. subscapular n. + thoracodorsal n. + L. subscapular n.; terminates as axillary n. + radial n.
  - – injury to U. trunk: 'waiter's tip'
  - – injury to L. trunk: 'claw hand'
- **Musculocutaneous n. (C5–7)**

- – arises from lateral cord
- – pierces coracobrachialis
- – lies between biceps brachii and brachialis
- – motor SS to flexor muscles on ant. arm + sensory SS to skin on lat. forearm
- **Boundaries of cubital fossa**
  - – roof: bicipital aponeurosis
  - – floor: brachialis, supinator
  - – sup. boundary: line between medial epicondyle and lateral epicondyle of humerus
  - – medial boundary: pronator teres
  - – lateral boundary: brachioradialis
- **Cubital fossa contents**
  - – tendon of biceps brachii (lat.)
  - – brachial a., radial a. and ulnar a.
  - – median n. (med.)
- **Median n. (C6–8, T1)**
  - – motor SS: all muscles in ant. compartments of FA (except flexor carpi ulnaris and medial half of flexor digitorum profundus) + three thenar m. + two lat. lumbricals
  - – sensory SS: skin over palmar surface of lat. three and a half fingers and lat. palm
- **Ulnar n. (C7–8, T1)**
  - – motor SS: all intrinsic muscles of hand (except thenar m. and two lat. lumbricals), flexor carpi ulnaris, medial half of flexor digitorum profundus in FA
  - – sensory SS: skin over palmar and dorsal surfaces of medial one and a half fingers and medial palm
- **Radial n. (C5–8, T1)**
  - – motor SS: all muscles in post. compartments of arm and FA
  - – sensory SS: skin over post. surface of arm and FA, lat. surface of arm, and dorsal lat. surface of hand
  - – deep branch (motor) and superficial branch (sensory)
  - – deep branch becomes post. interosseous n. after emerging between two heads of supinator m.
- Radiocarpal joint formed by radius, scaphoid and lunate bones
- Structures in palm (from superficial to deep):
  - – skin → palmar aponeurosis → sup. palmar arch of ulnar a. → median + ulnar n. → flexor digitorum superficialis → tendons of flexor digitorum profundus → lumbrical m. → deep palmar arch of radial a. → ulnar n. (deep branch) → adductor pollicis + dorsal interossei
- **Attachments of pronator teres**
  - – origin (humeral head): medial epicondyle
  - – origin (ulnar head): coronoid process
  - – insertion: lat. radius
  - – nerve SS: median n. (C6 and 7)

- function: pronate and flex forearm
- **Attachments of flexor carpi ulnaris**
  - origin (humeral head): medial epicondyle of humerus
  - origin (ulnar head): medial olecranon of ulna
  - insertion: pisiform, hamate, base of fifth metacarpal bone
  - nerve SS: ulnar n. (C7–T1)
  - function: flex and adduct wrist joint
- **Attachments of palmaris longus**
  - origin: medial epicondyle of humerus
  - insertion: flexor retinaculum
  - nerve SS: median n. (C6 and 7)
  - function: flex forearm and hand
- **Attachments of flexor carpi radialis**
  - origin: medial epicondyle of humerus
  - insertion: bases of second and third metacarpal bones
  - nerve SS: median n. (C6 and 7)
  - function: flex and abduct wrist joint
- **Attachments of flexor digitorum superficialis**
  - origin (humero-ulnar head): medial epicondyle of humerus and coronoid process
  - origin (radial head): oblique line of radius
  - insertion: tendons to middle phalanges of medial four fingers
  - nerve SS: median n. (C8, T1)
  - function: flex proximal interphalangeal joints of medial four fingers, metacarpophalangeal joints of medial four fingers and wrist joint
- **Attachments of flexor digitorum profundus (deep to flexor digitorum superficialis)**
  - origin: U. part of ulna
  - insertion: distal phalanges of medial four fingers
  - nerve SS: median n. (C8, T1), ulnar n. (C8, T1)
  - function: flex interphalangeal joints
- **Attachments of flexor pollicis longus**
  - origin: ant. radius and interosseous memb.
  - insertion: base of distal phalanx of thumb
  - nerve SS: median n. (C7 and 8) (ant. interosseous n.)
  - function: flex distal phalanx of thumb
- **Attachments of pronator quadratus**
  - origin: distal ant. ulna
  - insertion: distal ant. radius
  - nerve SS: medial n. (C7 and 8) (ant. interosseous n.)
  - function: pronation
- **Attachments of extensor indicis**
  - origin: dorsal surface of ulna
  - insertion: extensor hood of index finger
  - nerve SS: post. interosseous n. (C7 and 8)
  - function: extend index finger

- **Attachments of extensor pollicis longus**
  - origin: dorsal surface of ulna
  - insertion: dorsal base of distal phalanx of thumb
  - nerve SS: post. interosseous n. (C7 and 8)
  - function: extend interphalangeal joint of thumb
- **Attachments of extensor pollicis brevis**
  - origin: dorsal surface of radius
  - insertion: dorsal base of proximal phalanx of thumb
  - nerve SS: post. interosseous n. (C7 and 8)
  - function: extend metacarpophalangeal joint of thumb
- **Attachments of abductor pollicis longus**
  - origin: dorsal surface of ulna and radius
  - insertion: lat. base of first metacarpal bone
  - nerve SS: post. interosseous n. (C7 and 8)
  - function: abduct thumb
- **Attachments of brachioradialis**
  - origin: lat. supraepicondylar ridge of humerus
  - insertion: lat. distal radius
  - nerve SS: radial n. (C5 and 6)
  - function: flex elbow when forearm is pronated
- **Attachments of extensor carpi ulnaris**
  - origin: lat. epicondyle of humerus
  - insertion: medial surface of fifth metacarpal
  - nerve SS: post. interosseous n. (C7 and 8)
  - function: extend and adduct wrist
- **Attachments of extensor digiti minimi**
  - origin: lat. epicondyle of humerus
  - insertion: dorsal surface of little finger
  - nerve SS: post. interosseous n. (C7 and 8)
  - function: extend little finger
- **Attachments of extensor digitorum**
  - origin: lat. epicondyle of humerus
  - insertion: middle and distal phalanges of lat. four fingers
  - nerve SS: post. interosseous n. (C7 and 8)
  - function: extend lat. four fingers
- **Attachments of extensor carpi radialis brevis**
  - origin: lat. supraepicondylar ridge of humerus
  - insertion: dorsal base of first and second metacarpal bones
  - nerve SS: radial n. (deep branch) (C6 and 7)
  - function: extend and abduct wrist
- **Attachments of extensor carpi radialis longus**
  - origin: lat. supraepicondylar ridge of humerus
  - insertion: dorsal base of second metacarpal bone
  - nerve SS: radial n. (C6 and 7)
  - function: extend and abduct wrist
- **Contents of carpal tunnel**

- – four tendons of flexor digitorum superficialis
- – four tendons of flexor digitorum profundus
- – median n.
- – tendon of flexor pollicis longus (has own synovial sheath)
- – roof formed by flexor retinaculum
- **Carpal bones in the hand**
  - – (most distal and medial, in clockwise fashion) hamate → capitate → trapezoid → trapezium → scaphoid → lunate → pisiform
    (can be remembered by mnemonic Hamate Comes To Town, Shouting Loud to Pisiform)
- **Scaphoid**
  = most commonly fractured carpal bone
- **Anatomical snuffbox**
  - – best seen when thumb is extended and abducted
  - – lateral border = tendon of extensor pollicis brevis and tendon of abductor pollicis longus
  - – medial border = tendon of extensor pollicis longus
  - – floor = scaphoid + trapezium
  - – contents = radial a.
- **Thenar muscles (nerve SS = medial n.)**
  - – flexor pollicis brevis
  - – opponens pollicis
  - – abductor pollicis brevis
- **Attachments of flexor pollicis brevis**
  - – origin: tubercle of trapezium
  - – insertion: proximal phalanx of thumb
  - – nerve SS: recurrent branch of median n. (C8, T1)
  - – function: flex metacarpophalangeal joint of thumb
- **Attachments of opponens pollicis**
  - – origin: tubercle of trapezium
  - – insertion: lat. palmar surface of first metacarpal bone
  - – nerve SS: recurrent branch of median n. (C8, T1)
  - – function: medially rotate thumb
- **Attachments of abductor pollicis brevis**
  - – origin: tubercle of scaphoid and trapezium
  - – insertion: proximal phalanx of thumb
  - – nerve SS: recurrent branch of median n. (C8, T1)
  - – function: abduct metacarpophalangeal joint of thumb
- **Hypothenar muscles (nerve SS = ulnar n.)**
  - – flexor digiti minimi brevis
  - – opponens digiti minimi
  - – abductor digiti minimi
- **Attachments of flexor digiti minimi brevis**
  - – origin: hook of hamate
  - – insertion: proximal phalanx of little finger
  - – nerve SS: deep branch of ulnar n. (C8, T1)

- – function: flex metacarpophalangeal joint of little finger
- **Attachments of opponens digiti minimi**
  - – origin: hook of hamate
  - – insertion: medial surface of fifth metacarpal bone
  - – nerve SS: deep branch of ulnar n. (C8, T1)
  - – function: lat. rotate fifth metacarpal bone
- **Attachments of abductor digiti minimi**
  - – origin: pisiform
  - – insertion: proximal phalanx of little finger
  - – nerve SS: deep branch of ulnar n. (C8, T1)
  - – function: abduct metacarpophalangeal joint of little finger
- **Superficial palmar arch**
  - – mainly formed by ulnar a.
- **Deep palmar arch**
  - – mainly formed by radial a.

Common pathologies

Osteoarthritis
= inflammation of synovial joints
- Most commonly affects weight-bearing joints (hips and knees)
- Joint changes:
  - – focal loss of cartilage
  - – synovial hyperplasia
  - – formation of osteophytes
- Risk factors:
  - – gender (female)
  - – genetic predisposition
  - – occupational
  - – obesity
  - – pre-existing bone disease
  - – previous fractures
  - – gout
- Symptoms:
  - – restricted joint movement
  - – pain on movement
  - – pain on weight-bearing
- Signs:
  - – joint instability
  - – joint swelling
  - – crepitus on joint movement
  - – joint deformity
- Investigations:
  - – X-ray
  - – MRI

- Management:
  - physiotherapy
  - joint replacement

Rheumatoid arthritis (RA)
= chronic inflammation of joints
- Autoimmune disease
- Widespread synovitis
- Mostly affects females
- Associated with HLA-DR4
- Clinical features:
  - insidious onset
  - palpable rheumatoid nodules
  - arthritis of multiple joints
  - rheumatoid factor in plasma
  - pain and swelling of joints
- Extra-articular features:
  - pericarditis
  - anaemia
  - pulmonary nodules
  - splenomegaly
  - amyloidosis
- Investigations:
  - X-ray
  - functional assessment of joint function
- Management:
  - drugs (methotrexate, sulfasalazine)
  - physiotherapy

Colles' fracture
- Causes 'dinner-fork' deformity
- Affects distal radius (dorsal angulation and displacement)
- Most commonly caused by falling on outstretched hand

Carpal tunnel syndrome
- Compression of median nerve in carpal tunnel
- Risk factors:
  - family history
  - overuse
  - pregnancy
  - rheumatoid arthritis
  - oral contraceptive pill
- Symptoms:
  - paraesthesia of lateral three and a half fingers
  - thenar wasting (loss of control of fine movements of thumb)
- Investigations: nerve conduction studies

- Management: surgical decompression of flexor retinaculum

Malignant hyperpyrexia
- Due to defect in muscle ryanodine receptors
- Causes:
  - general anaesthesia (most common)
  - neuroleptics
- Signs:
  - high temperature
  - widespread rigidity of skeletal muscle
- Management:
  - dantrolene

12

Lower limb

- **Femur**
  - head (articulates with acetabulum)
  - greater and lesser trochanter (site for m. attachment)
  - intertrochanteric line joins greater and lesser trochanter
  - linea aspera (post. femur) (crest for m. attachment)
  - medial condyle (articulates with tibia)
  - lateral condyle (articulates with tibia)
- **Boundaries of femoral triangle**
  - medial border: medial adductor longus
  - superior border: inguinal ligament
  - lateral border: medial sartorius
- **Sciatic nerve**
  - arises from L4–S3
  - begins from midpoint between post. sup. iliac spine and ischial tuberosity
  - leaves pelvis through greater sciatic foramen below piriformis
  - descends on surface of adductor magnus
  - lies deep to hamstring muscles
  - terminal branches: common peroneal n. and tibial n.
  - motor SS: hamstring m. + leg m. + foot m.
  - sensory SS: lat. leg below knee
  - associated with inf. gluteal a.
  - to avoid sciatic nerve injections should be done at the U. outer quadrant of buttock
- **Common peroneal n. (L4 and 5, S1 and 2)**
  - runs around neck of fibula (vulnerable to damage)
  - terminal branches: superficial peroneal n. and deep peroneal n.
- **Superficial peroneal n.**
  - motor SS to peroneus longus and peroneus brevis
  - sensory SS to skin of lat. leg and dorsum of foot (excluding skin between first and second toes)

- **Deep peroneal n.**
  - motor SS to extensor hallucis longus, extensor digitorum longus, extensor digitorum brevis and tibialis anterior
  - sensory SS to skin between first and second toes
- **Tibial n. (L4, 5, S1–3)**
  - cutaneous branch given off in popliteal fossa = sural n. (SS lat. leg and foot)
  - motor SS to gastrocnemius, soleus, popliteus, flexor hallucis longus, flexor digitorum longus and tibialis posterior
- **Attachments of gluteus maximus**
  - origin: ilium + post. sacrum + sacrotuberous ligament + coccyx
  - insertion: gluteal tuberosity of femur (deep fibres) + iliotibial tract of fascia lata
  - nerve SS: inf. gluteal n. (L5–S2)
  - arterial SS: inf. gluteal a.
  - function: extend and lat. rotate femur
- **Attachments of gluteus medius**
  - origin: post. ilium between ant. and post. gluteal lines
  - insertion: greater trochanter of femur
  - nerve SS: sup. gluteal n. (L4–S1)
  - arterial SS: sup. gluteal a.
  - function: abduct and med. rotate femur; stabilise pelvis when walking
- **Attachments of gluteus minimus**
  - origin: post. ilium between ant. and inf. gluteal lines
  - insertion: ant. greater trochanter of femur
  - nerve SS: sup. gluteal n. (L4–S1)
  - arterial SS: sup. gluteal a.
  - function: abduct and medially rotate femur; stabilise pelvis when walking
- **Hip joint**
  - ball-and-socket joint
  - head of femur and acetabulum
- **Movements of hip joint**
  - adduction: adductor magnus, adductor longus and adductor brevis
  - flexion: iliacus, psoas major, rectus femoris, sartorius and pectineus
  - abduction: tensor fascia latae, gluteus medius and gluteus minimus
  - extension: gluteus maximus
  - medial rotation: gluteus medius and gluteus minimus
  - lateral rotation: gluteus maximus
- **Fascia lata**
  - fascia of thigh
  - attached post. to iliac crest and ant. to inguinal ligament
  - saphenous opening transmits long saphenous vein
- **Quadriceps femoris muscle**
  = rectus femoris + vastus lateralis + vastus medialis + vastus intermedius
  - (a) Rectus femoris
    - origin: ant. inf. iliac spine and edge of acetabulum

    – insertion: patella and tibial tuberosity
    – nerve SS: femoral n. (L2–4)
    – function: extend leg and flex thigh
  (b) Vastus lateralis
    – origin: lat. lip of linea aspera
    – insertion: patella and lateral condyle of tibia
    – nerve SS: femoral n. (L2–4)
    – function: extend leg and flex thigh
  (c) Vastus medialis
    – origin: intertrochanteric line
    – insertion: patella and medial condyle of tibia
    – nerve SS: femoral n. (L2–4)
    – function: extend leg and flex thigh
  (d) Vastus intermedius
    – origin: ant. and lat. shaft of femur
    – insertion: patella and tibial tuberosity
    – nerve SS: femoral n. (L2–4)
    – function: extend leg and flex thigh

- **Attachments of sartorius muscle**
  - origin: anterior superior iliac spine
  - insertion: medial tibia
  - nerve SS: femoral n. (L2–4)
  - function: flex thigh and leg
- **Attachments of obturator externus**
  - origin: obturator membrane
  - insertion: trochanteric fossa
  - nerve SS: obturator n. (L3 and 4)
  - function: laterally rotate thigh
- **Attachments of pectineus**
  - origin: pectineal line
  - insertion: post. femur
  - nerve SS: femoral n.
  - function: adduct and flex thigh
- **Attachments of gracilis**
  - origin: inf. pubic ramus
  - insertion: medial tibia
  - nerve SS: obturator n. (L2 and 3)
  - function: adduct thigh, flex leg
- **Attachments of adductor brevis**
  - origin: inf. pubic ramus
  - insertion: post. femur, linea aspera
  - nerve SS: obturator n. (L2 and 3)
  - function: adduct thigh
- **Attachments of adductor longus**
  - origin: body of pubis
  - insertion: medial linea aspera

- nerve SS: obturator n. (L2–4)
- function: adduct thigh
- **Attachments of adductor magnus**
  - origin (adductor part): ischiopubic ramus
  - origin (hamstring part): ischial tuberosity
  - insertion (adductor part): post. femur, linea aspera
  - insertion (hamstring part): adductor tubercle
  - nerve SS (adductor part): obturator n. (L2–4)
  - nerve SS (hamstring part): sciatic n. (L2–4)
  - function: adduct and medially rotate thigh
- **Adductor canal**
  - medial aspect of thigh
  - medially bounded by adductor longus
  - laterally bounded by vastus medius
  - roof formed by sartorius
- **Structures passing through adductor canal**
  - femoral a. + v.
  - saphenous n.
  - n. to vastus medius
- **Hamstring muscles**
  = biceps femoris + semitendinosus + semimembranosus
- **Attachments of biceps femoris**
  - origin (long head): ischial tuberosity
  - origin (short head): lat. lip of linea aspera
  - insertion: head of fibula
  - nerve SS: sciatic n. (L5–S2)
  - function: extend thigh, flex leg, laterally rotate thigh and leg
- **Attachments of semitendinosus**
  - origin: ischial tuberosity
  - insertion: medial tibia
  - nerve SS: sciatic n. (L5–S2)
  - function: extend thigh, flex leg, medially rotate thigh and leg
- **Attachments of semimembranosus**
  - origin: ischial tuberosity
  - insertion: post. tibial condyle
    nerve SS: sciatic n. (L4–S3)
  - function: extend thigh, flex leg, medially rotate thigh and knee
- **Blood SS to femoral head: medial circumflex femoral a.**
- Patella:
  - sesamoid bone
- Knee joint:
  - hinge joint
  - ligaments stabilising the joint
    - (a) ant. cruciate ligament: from ant. attachment on tibia → ascends
      post. to lateral wall of intercondylar fossa of femur
    - (b) post. cruciate ligament: from post. attachment on tibia → ascends

ant. to medial wall of intercondylar fossa of femur
  (c) medial collateral ligament (resists abduction)
  (d) lateral collateral ligament (resists adduction)
- **Movements of knee joint**
  - medial rotation: popliteus
  - flexion: biceps, semitendinosus, semimembranosus, gracilis, sartorius
  - extension: quadriceps femoris
- **Popliteal fossa**
  - structures within fossa (ant. to post.): popliteal a. (deepest structure), popliteal v., tibial n.
  - boundaries:
  sup. + lat.: biceps
  sup. + med.: semimembranosus + semitendinosus
  inf. + lat.: lat. head of gastrocnemius
  inf. + med.: med. head of gastrocnemius
- **Tibia (medial)**
  - medial condyle
  - lateral condyle
  - intercondylar eminence between medial and lateral condyles
  - tibial tuberosity (attachment site for patellar ligaments)
  - medial malleolus
- **Fibula**
  - head
  - neck (associated with common peroneal n.)
  - lateral malleolus (more distal than medial malleolus)
- **Attachments of tibialis anterior**
  - origin: lat. condyle of tibia + interosseous memb.
  - insertion: medial cuneiform + base of first metatarsal
  - nerve SS: deep peroneal n. (L4 and 5)
  - function: dorsiflex and invert foot
- **Attachments of extensor hallucis longus**
  - origin: medial fibula
  - insertion: base of distal phalanx of great toe
  - nerve SS: deep peroneal n. (L5, S1)
  - function: extend great toe, dorsiflex foot
- **Attachments of extensor digitorum longus**
  - origin: medial fibula
  - insertion: distal and middle phalanges of lateral four toes
  - nerve SS: deep peroneal n. (L5, S1)
  - function: extend lateral four toes, dorsiflex foot
- **Attachments of gastrocnemius**
  - origin: femoral epicondyles (med. + lat. heads)
  - insertion: Achilles' tendon → calcaneus
  - nerve SS: tibial n. (L4, 5, S1–3)
  - action: plantarflex ankle and flex knee
- **Attachments of plantaris (between soleus and gastrocnemius)**

- origin: lat. supracondylar line of femur
- insertion: Achilles' tendon → calcaneus
- nerve SS: tibial n. (L4 and 5, S1–3)
- action: plantarflex foot and flex knee
- **Attachments of soleus (under gastrocnemius)**
  - origin: post. fibular head and medial tibia
  - insertion: Achilles' tendon → calcaneus
  - action: plantarflex foot
- **Attachments of popliteus**
  - origin: post. proximal tibia
  - insertion: lat. femoral condyle
  - action: unlock knee joint (rotate femur laterally when tibia is fixed)
- **Attachments of flexor hallucis longus**
  - origin: post. fibula and interosseous memb.
  - insertion: distal phalanx of great toe
  - nerve SS: tibial n. (L4 and 5, S1–3)
  - action: flex great toe
- **Attachments of flexor digitorum longus**
  - origin: post. tibia
  - insertion: distal phalanges of lateral four toes
  - nerve SS: (L4 and 5, S1–3)
  - action: flex lateral four toes
- **Attachments of tibialis posterior**
  - origin: post. interosseous memb.
  - insertion: navicular and medial cuneiform
  - nerve SS: (L4 and 5, S1–3)
  - action: plantarflex and invert foot
- **Attachments of peroneus longus**
  - origin: fibular head
  - insertion: first metatarsal bone and first cuneiform bone
  - nerve SS: superficial peroneal n.
  - function: plantarflex and evert foot
- **Attachments of peroneus brevis**
  - origin: lateral fibula
  - insertion: fifth metatarsal bone
  - nerve SS: superficial peroneal n.
  - function: plantarflex and evert foot
- **Popliteal a.**
  - passes into post. compartment of leg between gastrocnemius and popliteus
  - divides into ant. and post. tibial a.
- **Ant. tibial a.**
  - pierces through interosseous membrane
  - SS: ant. compartment of leg
  - continues as dorsalis pedis a.
- **Post. tibial a.**

- – gives off peroneal a.
- – SS: lat. and post. compartments of leg
- – continues as medial and lateral plantar a.
- **Long saphenous vein**
  - – drains medial dorsum of foot
  - – passes ant. to medial malleolus
  - – pierces deep fascia 1 inch below inguinal ligament
  - – used for coronary bypass grafts
- **Short saphenous vein**
  - – drains lateral dorsum of foot
  - – passes post. to lateral malleolus
  - – pierces deep fascia over popliteal fossa
  - – closely associated with sural n. (branch of tibial n.)
- **Tarsal bones**
  - (a) Talus
    - – articulates with tibia superiorly
    - – articulates with calcaneus inferiorly
  - (b) Calcaneus
    - – largest tarsal bone
  - (c) Navicular
  - (d) Cuboid
  - (e) Cuneiforms
- **Ankle joint**
  - – synovial joint
  - – articular surfaces lined with hyaline cartilage
  - – between tibia and fibula of leg and talus of foot
  - – stabilised by deltoid ligament (medial) and lateral ligament
- **Movements of ankle joint**
  - – dorsiflexion: tibialis anterior
  - – plantarflexion: gastrocnemius, soleus, tibialis posterior
- **Subtalar joint**
  - – synovial joint
  - – between talus superiorly and calcaneus inferiorly
  - – stabilised by medial + lateral + posterior + interosseous talocalcaneal ligaments
- **Talocalcaneonavicular joint**
  - – synovial joint
  - – between talus superiorly + calcaneus inferiorly + navicular anteriorly
  - – stabilised by talonavicular ligament superiorly, interosseous talocalcaneal ligament posteriorly, and plantar calcaneonavicular ligament inferiorly
- **Calcaneocuboid joint**
  - – synovial joint
  - – between calcaneus posteriorly and cuboid anteriorly
  - – stabilised by long plantar ligament and plantar calcaneocuboid ligament inferiorly

- **Attachments of long plantar ligament**
  - ant.: bases of metatarsals
  - post.: inf. calcaneus
- **Tarsometatarsal joint**
  - between tarsal bones posteriorly and metatarsals anteriorly
- **Tarsal tunnel**
  - medial side of ankle
  - flexor retinaculum overlies it
- **Contents of tarsal tunnel (from post. to ant.)**
  - tendon of flexor hallucis longus
  - tibial n.
  - post. tibial a.
  - tendon of flexor digitorum longus
  - tendon of tibialis posterior
- **Metatarsal bones**
  - five in total
  - each has a head, shaft and base
- **Phalanges**
  - proximal phalanx
  - middle phalanx
  - distal phalanx
- **Medial longitudinal arch of foot**
  - calcaneus + talus + navicular + first to third cuneiform + first to third metatarsals
- **Lateral longitudinal arch of foot**
  - calcaneus + cuboid + fourth to fifth metatarsals
- **Short plantar ligament**
  - from plantar surface of calcaneus to cuboid
- **Plantar aponeurosis**
  - thickened deep fascia in sole of foot
  - from calcaneal tuberosity to toes
  - supports longitudinal arch of foot
- **Long plantar ligament**
  - from plantar surface of calcaneus to second to fourth metatarsals
- **Layers in the sole of foot (from superficial to deep)**
  - (a) (i) abductor hallucis
    - (ii) flexor digitorum brevis
    - (iii) abductor digiti minimi
  - (b) (i) quadratus plantae
    - (ii) lumbricals
  - (c) (i) flexor hallucis brevis
    - (ii) adductor hallucis
    - (iii) flexor digiti minimi brevis
  - (d) (i) dorsal interossei
    - (ii) plantar interossei

Common pathologies

Avascular necrosis (AVN) of femoral head
- Causes: fracture of neck of femur, idiopathic, steroid induced, pregnancy, sickle-cell anaemia
- Symptoms:
  - sudden onset of hip pain
  - pain worse at night
  - limited weight bearing
- Investigations:
  - X-ray (deformed femoral head and increased sclerosis)
  - MRI
- Management:
  - hip replacement

Damage to common peroneal n.
- Symptoms:
  - foot drop
  - inversion of foot
  - anaesthesia over ant. lat. leg and foot

Deep vein thrombosis (DVT)
- Risk factors:
  - trauma
  - immobility
  - oestrogen therapy
- Symptoms:
  - engorgement of superficial veins
  - tenderness of calf
  - swelling of calf
- Investigations: Doppler ultrasound scan
- Management:
  - low-molecular-weight heparin (LMWH)
  - warfarin

Varicose veins
= abnormally distended and tortuous veins
- Causes: incompetent valves connecting superficial and deep veins
- Risk factors:
  - prolonged standing
  - obesity
  - oral contraceptive pill
- Mostly occur in superficial saphenous veins
- May also occur in distal oesophagus and anorectal regions

Acute lower limb ischaemia
- Causes:
  - atherosclerotic emboli
  - aneurysm emboli
  - MI
  - atrial fibrillation
- Symptoms:
  - paralysis
  - paraesthesia
  - pallor
  - coldness
- Signs:
  - reduced sensation
  - reduced or absent pulses
  - compartment syndrome
- Investigations:
  - ankle/brachial pressure index (ABPI)
  - Doppler ultrasound scan
- Management:
  - heparin
  - warfarin

Chronic lower limb ischaemia
- Risk factors:
  - diabetes mellitus
  - hypercholesterolaemia
  - hypertension
  - smoking
- Symptoms:
  - intermittent claudication
- Signs:
  - cold, dry skin
  - ulceration
  - reduced or absent pulses
- Investigations:
  - ankle/brachial pressure index (ABPI)
  - Doppler ultrasound scan
- Management:
  - smoking cessation
  - percutaneous transluminal angioplasty
  - heparin
  - warfarin

Diabetic foot
- Causes:
  - diabetics susceptible to infection

- diabetics susceptible to atherosclerosis
- Symptoms:
  - painless necrosis of toes
  - ulceration at pressure points
  - painless penetrating ulcers due to infection
- Management:
  - oral antibiotics
  - excision of necrotic tissue

13

Back and central nervous system

- **Boundaries of intervertebral foramen (spinal nerves pass through)**
  - pedicles of two vertebrae
  - annulus fibrosus
  - facet joint
  - intervertebral disc
- **Cervical vertebrae (7)**
  - secondary curvature (concave post.)
  - C1 (atlas): X body, accommodates odontoid process of C2
  - C2 (axis): has odontoid process (dens) for rotation of head
  - C7: has palpable spinous process (vertebra prominens)
  - small and wide vertebral body
  - short, bifid spinous process
  - transverse process contains foramina
  - triangular-shaped vertebral canal
  - greatest range of movement in spine (flexion, extension, lat. flexion and rotation)
- Atlanto-occipital joint: flexion, extension, lateral flexion of head
  Atlanto-axial joint: rotation of head
- Supraspinous ligament = continuation of ligamentum nuchae
- **Thoracic vertebrae (12)**
  - primary curvature (concave ant.)
  - larger vertebral body than cervical vertebrae
  - long sharp spinous process
  - transverse process has facet for rib articulation
  - circular-shaped vertebral canal
  - rotation, lat. flexion only

- **Lumbar vertebrae (5)**
  - secondary curvature (concave post.)
  - large kidney-shaped vertebral body (for weight bearing)
  - short blunt spinous process
  - tapered thin transverse process
  - triangular-shaped vertebral canal
  - flexion, extension, lat. flexion
  - lumbar puncture usually performed at level L4/5 (spinal cord ends at L2)
- **Structures passed through when performing lumbar puncture**
  - skin → superficial fascia → supraspinous ligament → dura mater → arachnoid mater → subarachnoid space
- **Sacral vertebrae (5)**
  - primary curvature (concave ant.)
  - fused vertebral bodies
  - fused spinous process (forming median sacral crest)
  - U. part = sacral promontory
  - four ant. sacral foramina (transmit S1–4 ant. primary rami)
  - sacral hiatus (failure of lamina of S4 and 5 to fuse in midline)
  - no movement can occur
- **Intervertebral discs**
  - outer annulus fibrosis (thinner posteriorly) + inner nucleus pulposus
  - usually herniate posterolaterally through defect of annulus fibrosis → compress spinal n.
  - ant. relationships: ant. longitudinal lig.
  - post. relationships: post. longitudinal lig. (lies on ant. aspect of vertebral canal)
- **Intervertebral foramen**
  - ant. relationships: vertebral bodies
  - post. relationships: zygapophyseal joints
  - sup. and inf. relationships: vertebral pedicles
- **Attachments of trapezius muscle**
  - origin: ligamentum nuchae, supraspinous ligament up to T12
  - insertion: lateral third of clavicle, spine of scapula
  - nerve SS: spinal root of accessory n. (CNXI)
  - function: elevate and retract scapula and depress scapula
- **Attachments of latissimus dorsi**
  - origin: spinous processes of T7–12, post. third of iliac crest, inf. four ribs
  - insertion: floor of bicipital groove of humerus
  - nerve SS: thoracodorsal n. (C6–8)
  - function: adduct arm, medially rotate humerus, extend arm
- **Attachments of rhomboid minor**
  - origin: spinous processes of C7–T1
  - insertion: medial border of scapula above rhomboid major insertion
  - nerve SS: dorsal scapular n. (C5)
  - function: retract scapula
- **Attachments of rhomboid major**

- origin: spinous processes of T2–5
- insertion: medial border of scapula
- nerve SS: dorsal scapular n. (C5)
- arterial SS: deep branch of transverse cervical a.
- function: raise and retract scapula
- **Spinal cord**
  - developed from alar lamina and basal lamina separated by sulcus limitans
  - continuous with medulla oblongata
  - has cervical and lumbar enlargements
  - denticulate ligament connects pia mater to dura mater
  - ends at lower border of L1 as conus medullaris → continuous with a single layer of pia mater that attaches to first coccygeal vertebra (filum terminale)
  - subarachnoid space distal to conus medullaris = lumbar cistern
  - central canal contains CSF
  - H-shaped grey matter with ant. and post. horns joined centrally by grey commissure
  - lat. grey column present in thoracic and lumbar region (gives off preganglionic sympathetic fibres)
- **Meninges of spinal cord (outermost to innermost)**
  - dura mater
    - (i) outermost layer
    - (ii) internal to epidural space
  - arachnoid mater
  - pia mater (adheres tightly to spinal cord)
    - (i) vascular
    - (ii) forms denticulate ligaments on either side attaching to arachnoid mater and dura mater
    - (iii) separated from arachnoid by subarachnoid space (contains CSF)
  - inf. limit of subarachnoid space = S2
- **Arterial SS of spinal cord**
  - vertebral a. → ant. spinal artery and post. spinal arteries
  - ant. spinal artery runs in ant. median fissure
  - post. spinal arteries divide into two vessels each
  - radicular arteries
- **Spinal nerves (31 pairs)**
  - dorsal ramus = afferent; ventral ramus = efferent
  - dorsal ramus → medial and lat. (SS muscles and skin of back); contains dorsal root ganglion (DRG) (contains cell bodies)
  - ventral ramus (larger) → lat. cutaneous (post. and ant.) and ant. (medial and lat.) (SS body wall)
  - vertebral column grows faster than spinal cord → cord segments lie above corresponding vertebral bodies → in lumbosacral part dorsal and ventral nerve rootlets form cauda equina
- **Dorsal column system**
  - controls fine touch, proprioception and vibration sense

- skin, joints → dorsal horn → second-order neurons cross in medulla (cuneate nucleus/gracile nucleus) → spinal lemniscus in pons → medial lemniscus in midbrain → contralateral thalamus
- lesions above brainstem = deficits contralateral to lesion
- lesions in spinal cord = deficits ipsilateral to lesion
- **Spinothalamic tracts**
  - anterior spinothalamic tracts convey crude touch
  - lateral spinothalamic tracts convey temperature and sharp pain
  - skin → dorsal horn → second-order neurons cross in spinal cord near point of entry → contralateral thalamus
  - lesions in spinal cord = deficits contralateral to lesion
- **Corticospinal tract**
  - control skilled, voluntary movements
  - motor and premotor cortex → medullary pyramids → decussation of pyramids at lower medulla to descend as lateral corticospinal tract/ remain uncrossed and descend as anterior corticospinal tract and cross over at destination in ant. white commissure → alpha motor neurons
  - lateral corticospinal tract controls distal muscles
  - anterior corticospinal tract controls proximal muscles
- **Reticulospinal tract**
  - coordinates posture, fine control of voluntary movement, and spinal reflexes
  - reticular formation → cross at variable levels → alpha/gamma motor neurons
  - pontine reticular formation (excites extensor motoneurons)
  - medullary reticular formation (inhibits extensor motoneurons)
- **Tectospinal tract**
  - reflex postural movements governed by visual input
  - sup. colliculus (midbrain) → cross over near origin → alpha and gamma motor neurons
- **Vestibulospinal tract**
  - facilitates extensor muscles (increase tone in anti-gravity muscles) and inhibits flexor muscles
  - vestibular nuclei → does not cross over → alpha and gamma motor neurons
- **Neurons** = basic structural and functional units of nervous system
  - cell body + dendrites (towards cell body) + axons (away from cell body)
- **Neuroglia**
  - oligodendrocytes + astrocytes + microglia + ependymal cells + Schwann cells
  - oligodendrocytes form myelin in CNS
  - Schwann cells form myelin in PNS
- **White ramus communicans (WRC)**
  - connects spinal nerve to sympathetic ganglion
  - carries preganglionic fibres
- **Grey ramus communicans (GRC)**
  - connects sympathetic ganglion to spinal nerve
- **Sympathetic nerves**

- thoracolumbar outflow (T1– L2)
- short preganglionic and long postganglionic fibres
- dilate bronchi
- increase HR and BP
- T1–3 SS head and neck
- T4–6 SS UL
- T1–5 SS thoracic visceral organs (lungs, heart and oesophagus)
- T7–9 SS abdominal visceral organs
- T12– L2 SS LL
- **Parasympathetic nerves**
    - craniosacral outflow (CN 3, 7, 9 and 10)
    - long preganglionic and short postganglionic fibres
    - only distributed to head, neck, thoracic and abdominal viscera
    - constrict pupil
    - stimulate gland secretions
    - reduce HR and BP
- **Brain**
    - prosencephalon (forebrain) + mesencephalon (midbrain) + rhombencephalon (hindbrain)
    - telencephalon (cerebral hemispheres) + diencephalon (hypothalamus + thalamus + epithalamus + subthalamus) + mesencephalon (midbrain) + metencephalon (pons + cerebellum) + myelencephalon (medulla oblongata)
- **Arterial SS of brain**
    - circle of Willis = anastomosis between internal carotid a. and vertebral a.
    - internal carotid arteries (from common carotid a.)
    - vertebral arteries (from subclavian a.) → join on surface of pons to form basilar a. → post. cerebral arteries
- **Venous drainage of brain**
    - great cerebral v.
    - superficial middle cerebral v.
    - superior cerebral v.
- **Cerebral hemispheres**
    - frontal lobe (ant. cranial fossa)
    - temporal lobe (middle cranial fossa)
    - parietal lobe (above temporal lobe, between frontal and occipital lobes)
    - occipital lobe (above tentorium cerebelli)
    - central sulcus (between frontal and parietal lobes)
    - lateral sulcus
    - parieto-occipital sulcus
    - calcarine sulcus
    - three types of fibres
        - (a) projection fibres (from cerebral cortex to other parts of CNS) (e.g. corticospinal tracts)
        - (b) association fibres (connect one part of cerebral hemisphere to another part of the same cerebral hemisphere), e.g. long (connect

different lobes)/short (connect adjacent gyri) association fibres
- (c) commissural fibres (connect one part of cerebral hemisphere to same part of opposite cerebral hemisphere), e.g. corpus callosum
- **Basal ganglia (BG)**
  = grey matter masses in cerebral hemispheres
  - caudate nucleus + putamen + globus pallidus + subthalamic nucleus + substantia nigra
  - caudate nucleus + putamen + globus pallidus = corpus striatum
  - putamen + globus pallidus abut each other to form lentiform nucleus
  - major sites of input to BG = caudate + putamen
  - major sites of outflow of BG = globus pallidus
- Internal capsule runs between caudate nucleus and thalamus medially and lentiform nucleus laterally
- **Frontal lobe:** primary motor area (Brodmann's area 4) + prefrontal association area (ant.)
  - precentral sulcus ant. to precentral gyrus
  - precentral gyrus used for processing motor signals
- Broca's area (area 44, 45) controls motor speech (in inf. frontal gyrus)
- **Parietal lobe:** primary sensory area and sensory association area
  - postcentral gyrus used for processing sensory signals
- **Temporal lobe:** primary auditory area and auditory association area
  - Wernicke's area (area 22) controls language comprehension (input from Broca's area) (in sup. temporal gyrus)
  - hippocampus (memory)
- **Occipital lobe:** primary visual area (calcarine fissure) and visual association area
- **Insula** = floor of lateral sulcus
- **Dura mater of brain**
  - (a) Outer periosteal dura mater
    - in contact with internal table of diploe
    - rich vascular supply
  - (b) Inner meningeal dura mater
    - in contact with arachnoid
    - form falx cerebri + tentorium cerebelli + falx cerebelli + diaphragma sella
    - both layers attached to each other except in regions where they separate to form venous sinuses
    - arterial SS: middle meningeal a. (from maxillary a.)
- **Falx cerebri**
  - free border above corpus callosum
  - sup. border contains sup. sagittal sinus
  - inf. border contains inf. sagittal sinus
  - extends down into longitudinal fissure
  - attached to crista galli ant. and int. occipital protuberance post.
  - attached to tentorium cerebelli post.
- **Tentorium cerebelli**
  - has free margin (tentorial notch)

  - separates cerebellum from occipital lobe
  - tentorial notch encircles midbrain
  - fuses with falx cerebri
  - superior petrosal sinus along attachment to petrous bone
  - transverse sinus along attachment to occipital bone
- **Falx cerebelli**
  - between cerebellar hemispheres
  - attached to internal occipital crest
  - post. border contains occipital sinus
- **Diaphragma sella**
  - roof over hypophyseal fossa
  - penetrated by infundibulum of hypophysis
  - ant. and post. parts contain ant. and post. intercavernous sinuses
- **Brainstem**
  - diencephalon + midbrain + pons + medulla oblongata
- **Midbrain**
  - two cerebral peduncles (ant. part = crus cerebri; post. part = tegmentum; substantia nigra sandwiched between ant. and post. parts)
  - tectum: sup. + inf. colliculi = corpora quadrigemina
  - pineal gland between sup. colliculi
  - colliculi situated posteriorly
  - superior colliculus = reflex centre associated with visual pathway: receives fibres from lat. geniculate body
  - inferior colliculus = reflex centre associated with auditory pathway: receives fibres from cochlear nuclei, connects to med. geniculate body on each side
  - red nucleus receives efferent fibres from cerebellum → sends to thalamus and spinal cord
  - periaqueductal grey (PAG) around cerebral aqueduct: suppression of pain by producing endorphin
  - substantia nigra between PAG and red nucleus
- **Pons**
  - contains pontine nuclei
  - regulates and smooths out pattern of respiration
  - vertebral arteries join on surface to form basilar artery
- **Medulla oblongata**
  - inferior half is where decussation of pyramids occurs
  - primary respiratory, cardiovascular and vasomotor centre
- **Diencephalon**
  (a) Hypothalamus:
    - floor of third ventricle
    - mammillary bodies lie between cerebral peduncles
    - regulates body temperature, sleep and hunger
    - suprachiasmatic nucleus regulates circadian rhythm
    - connected to pituitary gland through infundibulum
    - forms releasing factors that control endocrine system

   (b) Thalamus:
- lat. walls of third ventricle
- central relay station for sensory nerve impulses travelling up from parts of body to cerebrum
- arterial SS: post. cerebral a.

   (c) Epithalamus:
- contains pineal body

- **Ventricles in the brain**
  - two lateral ventricles + third ventricle + fourth ventricle + cerebral aqueduct
  - two lateral ventricles connected via interventricular foramina of Monro
  - third ventricle connected to fourth ventricle by cerebral aqueduct
  - fourth ventricle drains into subarachnoid space via central foramen of Magendie and R. and L. foramina of Luschka

- **Pathway of flow of CSF from lateral ventricle**
  - lateral ventricle → interventricular foramen of Monro → third ventricle → cerebral aqueduct (midbrain) → fourth ventricle → subarachnoid space → arachnoid villi → superior sagittal sinus

- **Cerebellum**
  - occupies post. cranial fossa
  - ant. and post. and flocculonodular lobes
  - surface divided into folia
  - sup. thin layer of grey matter (cerebellar cortex)
  - white matter has multiple branches (arbor vitae)
  - two hemispheres connected centrally by vermis
  - connects to midbrain via superior cerebellar peduncles
  - connects to pons via middle cerebellar peduncles
  - connects to medulla via inferior cerebellar peduncles
  - nuclei contained = dentate n. (largest) + emboliform n. + globose n. + fastigial n.
  - arterial SS:
    - (i) ant. inf. cerebellar branches of basilar a.
    - (ii) sup. cerebellar branches of basilar a.
    - (iii) post. inf. cerebellar branches of vertebral a.

- **Reticular formation**
  - for arousal

- **Limbic system**
  = hippocampus + dentate gyrus + amygdala + cingulate gyrus

- **Mandible**
  - body meets ramus on either side at angle of mandible
  - mylohyoid line = oblique ridge of bone coursing backward to space behind third molar tooth (for attaching mylohyoid muscle) (separates mouth and neck)
  - U. border of body = alveolar part (for anchoring roots of teeth)
  - L. border of body = base (digastric fossa)
  - coronoid process (ant.): insertion for temporalis

- condyloid process (post.): articulates with temporal bone (temporomandibular joint)
- mental foramen below second premolar tooth
- structures passing through mental foramen = mental n. and mental a. + v.
- mandibular foramen leads to mandibular canal (transmits inferior alveolar n. + a.)
- **Temporomandibular joint**
  - only synovial joint in head
  - for mastication movements
  - covered with fibrocartilage
  - divided into two parts by fibrocartilaginous meniscus
  - lateral temporomandibular ligament limits movement of mandible posteriorly
  - sphenomandibular ligament: from spine of sphenoid → runs inferiorly → lingula of mandibular foramen
  - stylomandibular ligament: from styloid process → runs inferiorly → angle of mandible
  - movements:
    - (i) depression (contraction of lat. pterygoid + digastric + mylohyoid)
    - (ii) elevation (contraction of temporalis, masseter and medial pterygoid)
    - (iii) protraction (contraction of lateral pterygoid of both sides, and medial pterygoid)
    - (iv) retraction (contraction of post. fibres of temporalis)
    - (v) movement side to side (contraction of lat. and med. pterygoids)

Common pathologies

Myasthenia gravis
- Autoimmune disease
- Ab to ACh receptors in nicotinic postsynaptic neuromuscular junctions
- Symptoms:
  - ptosis
  - diplopia
  - muscle fatigue
  - muscle weakness after activity
- Investigations:
  - anti-ACh receptor antibodies
  - EMG
- Management:
  - immunosuppressive drugs (steroids)
  - anti-ACh inhibitors (pyridostigmine)

Duchenne muscular dystrophy
- X-linked disease

- Symptoms:
  - progressive muscle weakness
  - kyphoscoliosis
- Investigations:
  - raised creatinine kinase level
  - muscle biopsy
  - EMG

Osteoporosis

= reduction in bone-marrow density
- Bone resorption exceeds bone formation
- Causes:
  - menopause
  - Cushing's syndrome
  - rheumatoid arthritis (RA)
  - hyperthyroidism
  - hyperparathyroidism
  - drug induced (corticosteroids)
  - malabsorption of calcium
  - inflammatory bowel disease
  - hypogonadism
  - immobilisation
- Symptoms:
  - kyphosis
  - back pain
  - bone fracture
- Investigations:
  - blood tests (serum calcium levels)
  - bone densitometry
- Management:
  - physiotherapy
  - bisphosphonates (alendronate)
  - raloxifene (selective oestrogen-receptor modulator)
  - hormone replacement therapy (HRT) (associated with side-effects such as increased risk of cardiovascular diseases, thromboembolism)
  - parathyroid hormone

Osteomyelitis

= infection of bone marrow or bone
- Risk factors:
  - young children
  - septic arthritis
  - diabetes mellitus
  - sickle-cell anaemia

- Causes:
  - infectious spread through bloodstream (most commonly involves *Staphylococcus aureus*)
  - *Haemophilus influenzae* (in young children)
  - post-surgery infection
  - infection due to IV drug use
- Symptoms:
  - high temperature at metaphysis
  - inflammation
  - local tenderness
- Investigations:
  - blood tests (raised ESR and CRP)
  - bone biopsy and Gram stain
  - X-rays
  - MRI (cortical destruction)
- Management:
  - antibiotics
  - amputation of extremity

Paget's disease of bone
= increased bone remodelling
- Mostly affects axial skeleton
- Increased vascularity in affected bones
- Symptoms:
  - bone fractures
  - bone pain
    bone deformity
  - arthritis
- Investigations:
  - blood tests (increased ALP levels)
  - X-ray
  - bone scans
- Complications:
  - spinal cord compression
  - osteoarthritis
  - osteosarcoma
- Management:
  - bisphosphonates (alendronate)
  - calcitonin
  - painkillers
  - joint replacements

Rickets (in children) and osteomalacia (in adults)
- Cause:
  - malabsorption of vitamin D
  - low dietary intake of vitamin D

- - chronic renal failure
- - renal tubular acidosis
- • Clinical features:
  - - muscle pain
  - - pathological fractures
- • Investigations:
  - - blood tests (low serum 25-hydroxyvitamin D levels, raised ALP levels)
  - - bone biopsy
- • Management:
  - - vitamin replacement
  - - increase exposure to sunlight

Anencephaly
- • Failure of neural tube to close at cranial end

Spina bifida
- • Failure of neural tube to close at rostral end, and incomplete fusion of vertebral arches
- • Mostly at level L5/S1
- • Investigations:
  - - X-ray

Meningocoele
- • Herniation of arachnoid and dura mater through defect in vertebral column
- • Mostly occurs in lumbosacral region
- • Investigations:
  - - X-ray
  - - ultrasound scan
  - - MRI
- • Management:
  - - surgical excision

Meningomyelocoele
- • Protrusion of nerve roots and spinal cord through defect in vertebral column
- • Causes motor and sensory deficits below affected level
- • Investigations:
  - - X-ray
  - - ultrasound scan
  - - CT scan

Brown–Séquard syndrome
- • Complete hemisection of spinal cord
- • Contralateral impairment of pain and temperature sensation at level of hemisection (due to damage to spinothalamic tracts which have already

undergone decussation)
- Ipsilateral hemiplagia, impaired proprioception, and vibration sense below level of hemisection (damage to dorsal columns)
- Ipsilateral LMN signs at level of hemisection
- Ipsilateral UMN signs below level of hemisection (damage to lateral corticospinal tract)

Head contusions
- Coup injury (contusion in parts of brain underlying site of trauma)
- Contrecoup injury (contusion in parts of brain directly opposite site of trauma)

Secondary brain injury
- From complications that develop after primary brain injury (e.g. herniation of brain, cerebral hypoxia, oedema, intracerebral haemorrhage)

Herniation of brain
Cingulate herniation
- Cingulate gyrus herniates under falx cerebri
- Can lead to transtentorial herniation

Transtentorial herniation
- Supratentorial mass displaces temporal lobe
- Compression of CNIII → ipsilateral dilatation of pupil
- Compression of cerebral aqueduct → hydrocephalus
- Compression of midbrain → death
- Compression of cerebral peduncle → hemiparesis

Tonsillar herniation
- Herniation of cerebellar tonsils into foramen magnum
- Compression of medulla → respiratory compromise → death

Hydrocephalus
- Large amounts of CSF accumulated in brain ventricles/subarachnoid spaces
- Causes:
  - overproduction of CSF
  - obstruction to CSF flow
  - failure of CSF reabsorption
- Symptoms:
  - increased size of head (fetus)
  - features of increased ICP (headache, vomiting and papilloedema)
- Investigations: CT scan with contrast
- Management: drainage/shunting of ventricles

Berry aneurysm
- Congenital weakness of blood vessel in the brain

- Site: circle of Willis
- Usually occurs in hypertensive individuals
- Can lead to subarachnoid haemorrhage

Extradural haemorrhage
- Most commonly caused by fracture in temporal bone of skull
- Most commonly caused by damage to ant. division of middle meningeal a. (site of pterion)
- Symptoms:
  - 'lucid interval' before rapid deterioration
  - severe headache
  - fixed dilated pupil on side of injury
- Complication: increased intracranial pressure (ICP) by haematoma → pressure on underlying precentral gyrus with motor area
- Transtentorial herniation may take place
- Investigations: brain CT
- Management: evacuate blood by craniotomy

Subdural haemorrhage
- Acute cases mostly caused by trauma to front or back of head → displacement of brain antero-posteriorly
- Chronic cases mostly seen in the elderly (atrophy of brain renders bridging veins crossing subdural space vulnerable)
- Damage to sup. sagittal sinus occurs
- Blood accumulates between dura mater and arachnoid mater
- Clinical features develop gradually as venous blood is at low pressure (change in consciousness, and focal neurological signs such as limb weakness)
- Investigations:
  - brain CT/MRI
  - lumbar puncture
- Management: remove blood clot surgically
- Poor prognosis

Subarachnoid haemorrhage
- Risk factors:
  - oral contraceptive pill
  - smoking
  - ageing
- Causes:
  - rupture of aneurysm on circle of Willis (most common)
  - AV malformation
  - hypertensive haemorrhage
- Symptoms:
  - sudden onset of severe headache
  - nausea

- – vomiting
- – neck pain
- – may have diminished consciousness
- – focal neurological signs (hemiparesis, aphasia)
- – ocular haemorrhage
- Signs:
  - – photophobia
- Complications:
  - – hydrocephalus
  - – diabetes insipidus
- Investigations:
  - – brain CT
  - – lumbar puncture if CT is normal
  - – cerebral angiography
- Management:
  - – aneurysm: surgery
  - – AV malformation: conservative treatment

Intracerebral haemorrhage
- Formation of focal haematoma (space-occupying lesion)
- Most commonly occur in patients with chronic HT
- Other risk factors:
  - – ageing
  - – arteriovenous malformation
  - – anticoagulant treatment
- Most commonly due to rupture of branch of middle cerebral artery
- Symptoms:
    hemiplagia of opposite side of body
  - – loss of consciousness
  - – signs of raised ICP (headache, vomiting, decreased level of consciousness, papilloedema)
- Complications:
  - – dysphagia
  - – epilepsy
  - – deep vein thrombosis
  - – pressure sores
  - – urinary tract infection
  - – chest infection
- Investigations:
  - – brain CT/MRI
- Management:
  - – decompression of haematoma
  - – ischaemic stroke: thrombolysis
  - – haemorrhagic stroke: lower blood pressure (give diuretics)
- Reason for not performing lumbar puncture when increased ICP is suspected:

- withdrawing CSF displaces cerebral hemispheres through opening in tentorum cerebelli
- medulla and cerebellum will herniate through foramen magnum

Broca's aphasia (expressive aphasia)
- Comprehension of spoken language remains intact
- Ability to repeat spoken language is impaired
- Mostly caused by stroke on RHS of brain
- Patient is aware of deficit
- Investigations: CT scan

Wernicke's aphasia
- Speech remains fluent
- Ability to repeat and comprehend spoken language is impaired
- Mostly caused by stroke
- Patient is unaware of deficit

Neuroglial tumours
- Glioblastoma (highly malignant)

Encephalitis
= inflammation of parenchymal tissue in brain
- Causes:
  - viral infection (herpes simplex, mumps, Coxsackie, Epstein–Barr virus) (most common cause)
  - bacterial infection (*Staphylococcus aureus*)
  - parasitic infection
- Symptoms:
  - drowsiness
  - nausea
  - vomiting
  - headache
  - stiff neck
  - high fever
  - focal neurological signs
- Investigations:
  - blood tests (viral serology)
  - CSF analysis
  - CT of brain
  - MRI
  - brain tissue biopsy

Meningitis
= inflammation of meninges
- Pachymeningitis = inflammation of dura mater

- Leptomeningitis = inflammation of pia mater/arachnoid mater
- Causes:
  - bacterial infection (*Neisseria meningitidis*, *Staphylococcus aureus*, *Mycobacterium tuberculosis*)
  - viral infection (enteroviruses, herpes simplex, mumps, HIV)
  - fungal infection (*Candida*)
- Symptoms:
  - irritability (in children)
  - high fever and chills
  - acute onset of headache
  - stiff neck
  - photophobia
  - nausea
  - vomiting
  - drowsiness
  - seizures
- Signs:
  - Kernig's sign
- Investigations:
  - lumbar puncture
  - Gram stain of CSF
  - blood culture
  - PCR (viral cause)
  - CT scan
  - CSF fluid profiles

Bacterial meningitis
- Raised neutrophil count
- Reduced glucose levels
- Raised protein levels

Viral meningitis
- Raised lymphocyte count
- Raised protein levels

Fungal meningitis
- Cloudy appearance
- Reduced glucose levels
- Raised lymphocyte count
- Raised protein levels
- Management:
  - ampicillin and cefotaxime (in children)
  - penicillin (in adults)
- Complications:
  - hydrocephalus
  - seizures

Seizures
= convulsions in association with EEG changes resulting from abnormal electrical activity of cerebral neurons

Generalised seizures
- Bilateral abnormal electrical activity
- Loss of consciousness:
  - absence seizures = petit mal seizures (brief episodes of impaired consciousness lasting a few seconds)
  - tonic–clonic seizures = grand mal seizures (sudden onset of loss of consciousness with tonic extension of back and extremities, repetitive clonic movements and postictal muscle ache)
  - myoclonic seizures
  - tonic seizures

Partial seizures
- Localised seizure:
  - simple (no loss of consciousness)
  - complex (loss of consciousness)
- Causes:
  - acute hypoxia
  - alcohol withdrawal
  - cerebrovascular disease (arteriovenous malformation)
  - drug abuse (e.g. cocaine)
  - pyrexia
  - encephalitis
  - cerebral haemorrhage
  - cerebral infarction
  - cerebral abscess
  - neurodegenerative disorders
  - intracranial tumour
  - metabolic abnormalities (hypoglycaemia, hypocalcaemia)
  - HIV infection
- Investigations:
  - blood tests (calcium levels)
  - EEG
  - CT scan
  - MRI
- Management: anti-epileptic drugs

Status epilepticus
= prolonged seizure without regaining of consciousness
- Medical emergency
- Management:
  - protect airway
  - IV diazepam

Upper motor neuron (UMN) lesion
= lesion in neural path above ant. horn cells at spinal cord (corticospinal tract) (usually seen in stroke)
- Weakness in extensors of UL + flexors of LL; spasticity in unopposed muscle groups
- Loss of fine control of finger movements
- Positive Babinski sign
- Hyperreflexia
- Clasp-knife rigidity
- Spasticity
- Severe paralysis

Lower motor neuron (LMN) lesion
= lesion in neural path from ant. horn cells at spinal cord to muscles
- Muscle wasting
- Flaccidity
- Paralysis
- Fasciculations
- Hypotonia
- Hyporeflexia

Hemiplegia
= paralysis of one side of body

Paraplegia
= paralysis of both lower limbs

Quadriplegia
= paralysis of all four limbs

Huntington's disease
- Autosomal dominant disease
- Pathological basis: loss of GABA-ergic neurons in striatum → increased dopamine release
- Symptoms:
    - Huntington's chorea (uncontrolled movements)
    - irritability
    - depression
    - cognitive impairment
    - loss of fine manual skills
- Investigations:
    - DNA testing
    - CT scan (atrophy of caudate nucleus)
    - MRI
- Management:

- genetic counselling
- dopamine antagonists

Narcolepsy
- Symptoms:
  - sporadic episodes of uncontrollable sleep
  - cataplexy (sudden transient loss of muscle tone)

Multiple sclerosis (MS)
- Chronic neurological condition with progressive demyelination of white matter in brain and spinal cord (oligodendrocytes)
- Autoimmune disease
- Characterised by periods of remission and relapse, eventually leading to disability
- Pathology:
  - chronic inflammatory cells
  - myelin damaged with sparing of axons
- Symptoms:
  - paraplegia
  - visual disturbances, e.g. blurred vision (optic neuritis), diplopia
  - vertigo
  - focal numbness
  - sensory disturbances
  - recurrent facial palsy
  - incontinence
- Signs:
  - impaired visual acuity
  - swollen optic disc on fundoscopy
  - spasticity
- Complications:
  - spasticity
  - ataxia
  - fatigue
  - urgency and frequency
- Investigations:
  - MRI of brain and spinal cord
  - CSF examination (raised immunoglobins, oligoclonal bands)
- Management:
  - high-dose methylprednisolone
  - β-interferon (reduces rate of relapse)

14

Sensory organs

- **Extrinsic muscles of the eye**
  - sup. + inf. rectus; lat. + med. rectus; sup. + inf. oblique
- **Attachments of sup. rectus**
  - origin: sup. part of common tendinous ring
  - insertion: sup. ant. part of pupil
  - nerve SS: CNIII (sup. branch)
  - function: elevation and adduction of pupil
- **Attachments of inf. rectus**
  - origin: inf. part of common tendinous ring
  - insertion: inf. ant. part of pupil
  - nerve SS: CNIII (inf. branch)
  - function: depression and adduction of pupil
- **Attachments of lat. rectus**
  - origin: lat. part of common tendinous ring
  - insertion: lat. ant. part of pupil
  - nerve SS: CNVI
  - function: abduction of pupil
- **Attachments of med. rectus**
  - origin: lat. part of common tendinous ring
  - insertion: med. ant. part of pupil
  - nerve SS: CNIII (inf. branch)
  - function: adduction of pupil
- **Attachments of sup. oblique**
  - origin: body of sphenoid bone
  - insertion: lat. post. part of pupil
  - nerve SS: CNIV
  - function: depression and abduction of pupil

- **Attachments of inf. oblique**
  - origin: medial orbit
  - insertion: lat. post. part of pupil
  - nerve SS: CNIII (inf. branch)
  - function: elevation and abduction of pupil
- **Attachments of levator palpebrae superioris**
  - origin: lesser wing of sphenoid bone
  - insertion: superior tarsal plate, skin of U. lid also contains smooth muscle fibres that attach to superior tarsal plate
  - nerve SS: oculomotor n.
  - smooth muscle SS: sympathetic fibres
  - function: raise U. eyelid
- **Lacrimal apparatus**
  - lacrimal gland → excretory ductules → superior fornix of conjunctival sac → sup./inf. lacrimal papilla → punctum → sup./inf. lacrimal canaliculi → lacrimal sac → nasolacrimal duct → inf. meatus of nose
- **Tarsal glands (contained in tarsal plate)**
  - open behind eyelashes
  - function: prevent overflow of tears, keep closed eyelids airtight
- **Sclera**
  - dense connective tissue
  - attached to choroid internally
- **Choroid**
  - vascular pigmented layer
  - attached to retina internally
- **Iris**
  - dilator pupillae (dilates pupil)
  - sphincter pupillae (constricts pupil)
  - attached to ciliary body posteriorly
- **Retina**
  - outer pigmented layer
  - inner nervous layer
  - fovea centralis = most light-sensitive area, 4 mm lateral to optic disc
  - rods (contain pigment rhodopsin) and cones
  - rods: high convergence to ganglion cells (many rods synapse on one bipolar cell) → less acuity but greater sensitivity
- **Photo-transduction pathway**
  - light → phosphodiesterase activated → intracellular cGMP levels decrease → sodium channels close → photoreceptors hyperpolarise
- **Visual pathway**
  - optic n. → lateral geniculate body of thalamus → visual cortex
- **Ciliary body** = ciliary process + ciliary muscle
  Ciliary process: produces aqueous humour
  Ciliary muscle: changes lens shape (accommodation)
- Ant. chamber contains aqueous humour
  Post. chamber contains vitreous humour

- **Paranasal sinuses** (air spaces in skull communicating with nasal cavity)
  - (a) maxillary sinus
  - (b) ethmoid sinuses (ant. + middle + post.)
    - – lie between orbits and nasal cavity
  - (c) frontal sinus
  - (d) sphenoid sinus
- **Drainage of paranasal sinuses**
  - – maxillary sinus: hiatus semilunaris
  - – sphenoid sinus: sphenoethmoidal recess
  - – frontal sinus: middle nasal meatus
  - – post. ethmoidal sinus: sup. nasal meatus
  - – middle ethmoidal sinus: ethmoid bulla (middle nasal meatus)
  - – ant. ethmoidal sinus: hiatus semilunaris
- **Walls of nasal cavity**
  - (a) roof
    - – nasal bone
    - – frontal bone
    - – cribriform plate of ethmoid bone
    - – body of sphenoid
  - (b) medial wall
    - – nasal septum
  - (c) lateral wall
    - – nasal bone
    - – maxilla
    - – lacrimal bone
    - – ethmoid bone
    - – perpendicular plate of palatine bone
    - – medial pterygoid plate of sphenoid bone
  - (d) floor
    - – horizontal plate of palatine bone
    - – palatine process of maxilla
- **Nasal septum**
  - – vomer and perpendicular plate of ethmoid bone
  - – sensory SS by nasociliary n. (branch of CNV_1)
- Lateral wall of nasal cavity contains superior + middle + inferior nasal conchae with meatus below each concha
- Space above sup. nasal conchae = sphenoethmoidal recess
- **Arterial SS to nasal cavity**
  - – sphenopalatine a. (from maxillary a.)
  - – ant. ethmoidal a. (from opthalmic a.)
- **Waldeyer's ring**
  = circle of protective lymphatic tissue at the U. ends of respiratory and alimentary tracts
  - – lingual tonsil (midline) (under post. tongue)
  - – palatine tonsils (around oropharynx)

- – tubal tonsils (around openings of auditory tube)
- – pharyngeal tonsil (midline) (in nasopharynx)
- **External ear**
  - – pinna and ext. auditory canal
- **Pinna (elastic cartilage)**
  - – channels sound waves into external auditory meatus
  - – tragus (ant.)
  - – intertragic notch
  - – antitragus
  - – lobule
- **Middle ear**
  - – contains three ossicles: malleus (in contact with tympanic membrane) + incus + stapes (in contact with oval window), which transmit sound vibrations between tympanic membrane and inner ear
  - – soundwaves travel from tympanic membrane → malleus → incus → stapes → oval window and round window
  - – malleus attaches to tensor tympani muscle
  - – stapes attaches to stapedius muscle
  - – relationships:
    medial: round window and oval window
    ant.: Eustachian tube
    lateral: tympanic membrane
  - – Eustachian tube connects nasopharynx to middle ear
- **Inner ear**
  - – acoustic apparatus: cochlea (filled with perilymph)
  - – cochlea: organ of Corti (sends nerve impulses to brainstem through CN VIII)
  - – vestibular apparatus: vestibule and semicircular canals
  - – vestibule: utricle and saccule (hair cells embedded in otoliths)
  - – muscles: stapedius muscle and tensor tympani (damp down high-frequency sounds)
- **Innervation of inner ear muscles**
  - – stapedius (chorda tympani CN VII)
  - – tensor tympani (CN V_3)
- **Auditory pathway**
  - – cochlear hair cells → spiral ganglion of cochlear n. → CN VIII → cochlear nuclei (medulla) → synapse in superior olivary nuclei → lateral leminisci → inferior colliculi → medial geniculate body (thalamus) → primary auditory cortex
- **Pharyngotympanic tube:** connects middle ear and nasopharynx
- **Tongue**
  - – circumvallate papillae (ant. to sulcus terminalis)
  - – foliate papillae
  - – fungiform papillae
  - – filiform papillae
- Sulcus terminalis lies between post. third of tongue and ant. two-thirds of tongue

- Foramen caecum = U. end of thyroglossal duct
- **Extrinsic muscles of tongue (move tongue)**
  - Palatoglossus
  - Styloglossus
  - Genioglossus
  - Hyoglossus
- **Intrinsic muscles of tongue (alter shape of tongue)**
  - longitudinal bundles
  - transverse bundles
  - vertical bundles
- **Innervation of tongue**
  (a) Oral part (ant. two-thirds)
    - sensory SS from lingual n. (CN V_3)
    - taste from chorda tympani (CN VII)
  (b) Pharyngeal part (post. third):
    - sensory SS + taste from glossopharyngeal n. + vagus n. (CN IX+ CN X)
- **Arterial SS of tongue**
  - lingual a. (ext. carotid a.)
  - ascending pharyngeal a.
  - tonsillar branch of facial a.
- **Lymphatic drainage of tongue**
  - tip of tongue: submental lymph nodes
  - ant. two-thirds of tongue: submandibular lymph nodes and deep cervical nodes
  - post. third of tongue: deep cervical nodes
- **Lingual a.**
  - between genioglossus medially and hyoglossus laterally
- **Lingual n. (CN V3)**
  - joined by chorda tympani (CN VII)
- **Hypoglossal n.**
  - travels with lingual v.
  - between hyoglossus medially and mylohyoid laterally
  - overlies loop on lingual a.
- **Sublingual gland**
  - opens along sublingual folds at base of frenulum
  - between genioglossus and myohyoid
- **Lymphatic drainage**
  - ant. two-thirds drain to jugulo-omohyoid node (through submandibular nodes)
  - post. third drains to jugulo-digastric node (also drains lymph from orophraynx and palatine tonsil)
- **Nervous pathway for taste sensation**
  - CN VII, IX and X → solitary n. (medulla) → solitary tract → ipsilat. to ventral post. medial nucleus (thalamus) → taste cortex (insula) → hypothalamus and limbic system

Common pathologies

Astigmatism
- Uneven curvature of cornea/lens in vertical and horizontal planes
- Management:
  - cylindrical lens

Iritis
- Inflammation of iris
- Causes:
  - ankylosing spondylitis (AS)
  - syphilis
  - HSV
  - trauma
- Symptoms:
  - reduced visual acuity
- Complications:
  - cataracts
- Management:
  - topical steroids

Myopia
- Elongated eyeball
- Symptoms:
  - blurred distant vision
- Complications:
  - retinal detachment
- Management:
  - concave lens

Hyperopia
- Shortened eyeball
- Symptoms:
  - blurred near vision
- Complications:
  - angle-closure glaucoma
- Management:
  - convex lens

Primary open-angle glaucoma
- Most common type of glaucoma
- Risk factors:
  - myopia
  - hypertension
  - age > 40 years
  - family history

- anaemia
- Symptoms:
  - progressive loss of peripheral vision
  - cupping of optic disc
  - loss of central vision (in later stages)
- Management:
  - topical cholinergics
  - topical adrenergics
  - topical carbonic anhydrase inhibitors

Secondary open-angle glaucoma
- Traumatic glaucoma
- Steroid-induced glaucoma (corticosteroid use)

Primary angle-closure glaucoma
- Risk factors:
  - pupil dilation (applied anticholinergics)
  - age > 70 years
  - family history
- Symptoms:
  - red eye
  - halo surrounding lights
  - reduced visual acuity
  - nausea
  - vomiting
- Management:
  - pilocarpine
  - systemic carbonic anhydrase inhibitors
  - systemic hyperosmotic agents (mannitol)
  - surgery
- Complications:
  - irreversible loss of vision

Cataract
- Clouding of lens
- Most common cause of reversible blindness
- Causes:
  - ageing
  - congenital
  - diabetes mellitus
  - hypocalaemia
  - drug induced (corticosteroids)
  - uveitis
- Symptoms:
  - gradual but painless loss of vision
- Management:

- incise lens
- remove cloudy core and provide artificial lens

Papilloedema
- Caused by increased intracranial pressure

Bitemporal hemianopsia
- Blindness in temporal half of visual field in each eye
- Mostly caused by lesion affecting optic chiasm, such as pituitary tumour

Age-related macular degeneration
- Causes visual impairment
- Deposition of drusen over macula
- More common in females
- Risk factors:
  - smoking
  - ageing
  - family history
- Symptoms:
  - blurred central vision
  - painless loss of vision
- Investigations:
  - fluorescein angiography
- Management:
  - laser photocoagulation (if neovascularisation occurs)
  - photodynamic therapy (PDT)

Hypertensive retinopathy
- Keith–Wagner classification:
  - grade I: arteriosclerosis occurs; a. with shiny walls (copper wiring)
  - grade II: AV nipping (narrowing of arterioles when crossing v.)
  - grade III: flame haemorrhages, retinal oedema, cottonwool spots, macular star
  - grade IV: papilloedema

Diabetic retinopathy
Background retinopathy
- Cottonwool spots
- Dot and blot haemorrhages
- Hard exudates
- Microaneurysms

Pre-proliferative retinopathy
- Arteriolar narrowing
- Multiple cottonwool spots
- Intraretinal microvascular abnormalities (IRMA)

- Macular oedema

Proliferative retinopathy
- Neovascularisation around disc (NVD)
- Preretinal haemorrhage
- Urgent management needed

Infection of frontal sinus
- In close proximity to frontal lobe of brain → may cause formation of frontal lobe abscess

Otitis media
= acute inflammation of middle ear
- Causes:
  - viral infection
- Symptoms:
  - conductive deafness
  - severe pain
- Complications:
  - spread to mastoid bone
- Management:
  - antibiotics

Conductive deafness
- Due to lesion in external auditory meatus, tympanic membrane or middle ear structures
- Possible causes:
  - neoplasm in external auditory canal
  - obstruction of external auditory meatus by foreign body
  - perforation of tympanic membrane

Sensorineural deafness
- Due to lesion in CN VIII/inner ear
- Possible causes:
  - fracture of temporal bone
  - acoustic neuroma
  - viral infection
  - ototoxic drugs
  - damaged hair cells in organ of Corti

Ménière's disease
- Symptoms:
  - vertigo
  - tinnitus
  - deafness
- Disorder of endolymph system

15

Integumentary system

- **Skin**
- epidermis + dermis
    - (a) Epidermis:
        - derived from ectoderm
        - stratified squamous epithelium
        - avascular
        - (from outermost to innermost): stratum corneum → stratum lucidum → stratum granulosum → stratum spinosum → stratum basale (contains melanin)
        - keratinocytes (synthesise structural proteins)
        - Merkel cells
        - Langerhans cells (dendritic cells that present antigens to lymphocytes)
        - melanocytes
    - (b) Basement membrane
    - (c) Dermis:
        - derived from mesoderm
        - vascular layer
        - fibroblasts
        - blood vessels
        - nerves
        - sweat glands
        - hair follicles
- **Sweat glands**
    - (a) Apocrine glands
        - open into hair follicles
        - found in axilla, groin and anal region
    - (b) Eccrine glands
        - open on to surface of skin

– regulate body temperature
- **Sebaceous glands**
  - secrete sebum into hair follicles
  - lubricate hair and skin
  - sebaceous cyst forms when outlet is blocked completely

Common pathologies

Herpes zoster
- Infection caused by varicella zoster virus
- Most commonly occurs in thoracic region
- Risk factors:
  - immunosuppression
  - age
- Symptoms:
  - pain
  - fever
  - vesicles
- Signs: vesicular rash along dermatome distribution
- Management:
  - analgesics
  - acyclovir

Psoriasis
= chronic inflammatory condition of the skin
- Increased cell proliferation
- Risk factors: family history
- Pathological features: irregular thickening of epidermis
- Clinical features:
  - erythematous skin
  - onycholysis
- Management:
  - topical corticosteroids
  - UV radiation
  - oral retinoids

Eczema (also known as dermatitis)
= inflammatory condition of the skin
- Clinical features:
  - scale formation
  - dry skin
  - oedema in epidermis (spongiosus)
  - vesicles
  - itchiness
- Complications:

- – secondary infection
- Management:
  - – topical corticosteroids
  - – barrier creams
  - – avoid contact with irritants

Systemic lupus erythematosus (SLE)
= multi-system autoimmune inflammatory condition of connective tissue
- Production of autoantibodies
- Clinical features:
  - – fever
  - – cranial n. lesions
  - – myalgia
  - – arthritis of joints
  - – glomerulonephritis
  - – 'butterfly rash' on face
  - – purpura
  - – painful oral ulcers
  - – pleurisy
  - – pneumonitis
  - – pericarditis
  - – anaemia
  - – palmar erythema
  - – splinter haemorrhage
- Investigations:
  - – antinuclear antibodies
  - – raised levels of CRP and ESR
- Management:
  - – high-dose corticosteroids (acute conditions)
  - – NSAIDs
  - – analgesics

Marfan's syndrome
= disorder of connective tissue
- Autosomal dominant disorder
- Clinical features:
  - – dislocated lenses
  - – long arms, legs and fingers
  - – mitral valve prolapse
  - – aortic aneurysm
  - – aortic dissection
  - – tall thin body
- Investigations:
  - – CXR (aortic aneurysm)
  - – echocardiogram (mitral regurgitation)
- Management:

- beta-blockers
- aortic root replacement

Basal-cell carcinoma (BCC)
- Malignant neoplasm of basal cells
- Commonly occurs on face
- Cause: UV exposure
- Symptoms:
  - pearly nodule with ulcerated centre
  - scaly plaques
- Management:
  - cryotherapy
  - surgical excision

Squamous-cell carcinoma (SCC)
- Malignant neoplasm of keratinocytes
- Causes:
  - UV radiation
  - chemical carcinogens
  - ionising radiation
- Symptoms:
  - ulcerated plaque with scale
- Management:
  - surgical excision

Malignant melanoma
- Tumour of melanocytes
- Most common cause: excessive exposure to sunlight
- Clinical features:
  - asymmetrical
  - variable pigmentation
  - irregular border
  - enlargement
  - irregular elevation
- Management: excision

Index

Printed and bound by CPI Group (UK) Ltd, Croydon, CR0 4YY

23/10/2024

01777665-0012